CALLED TO CARE

CALLED
to CARE

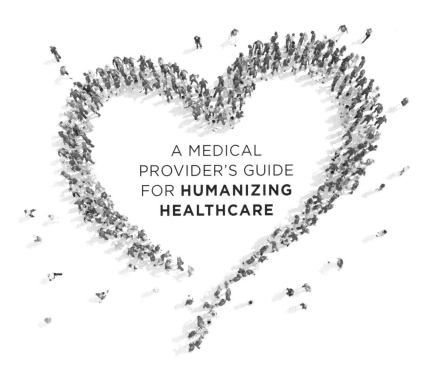

A MEDICAL
PROVIDER'S GUIDE
FOR **HUMANIZING
HEALTHCARE**

DR. LAURENCE N. BENZ,
PT, DPT, OCS, MBA, MAPP

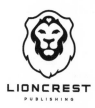

LIONCREST
PUBLISHING

CALLED TO CARE

A Medical Provider's Guide for Humanizing Healthcare

ISBN 978-1-5445-1489-5 *Hardcover*

  978-1-5445-1488-8 *Paperback*

  978-1-5445-1487-1 *Ebook*

  978-1-5445-1490-1 *Audiobook*

FIRST EDITION

This book is dedicated to my partners and teammates at Confluent Health. They demonstrate through actions what this book espouses in words. Also, to Patty, Aaron, Angela, Lauren, Donald, Jonathan, Levi, Cassie, and Samson. Because you were Called to Care for me, and that has made all the difference.

CONTENTS

PREFACE

As this book awaits publication, we are in the middle of fighting the novel coronavirus (COVID-19) across the globe. This has brought an unprecedented focus on healthcare and, in particular, public health, prevention, and the realization that a virus we cannot see can impart unforeseen sickness and fatalities. There are visuals of first responders and healthcare workers fighting at the front lines for people's lives. Formerly abstract terms like national emergency, pandemic, shelter at home, medical supply shortages, antibody testing, N95 masks, and mobile hospitals have real daily meaning. Many workers are deemed "essential," meaning they conduct a range of operations and services that are critical to the continued viability of our infrastructure as guided by the Department of Homeland Security acting via the Cybersecurity and Infrastructure Security Agency (CISA). Among these essential workers are the physical therapists who are part of the company I lead. It is fair to say, our lives have dramatically altered and will be changed by this in many ways, some permanent.

We are seeing unprecedented compassion, concern, and sympathy driving us to take action. For example, the US Congress bipartisan support of the Families First Coronavirus Response Act and CARES Act, which both passed and were signed by the president in record time. A significant number of states have passed legislation that relaxes and enhances unemployment filings. Health insurance companies have come together to waive co-pays and fully pay for any COVID-19 treatments. Thirty million-plus Americans without any health insurance have been given comfort that if they get COVID-19 their cost will be paid directly to the hospitals providing treatment. Government regulations regarding patient record keeping and even parts of HIPAA have been waived. Medical students in certain parts of the country graduated early to help fight and keep elderly and other vulnerable people at home. There is significant relief of mortgages, incredible generosity towards workers on the front lines, and highlighting of physicians and others as both warriors and heroes. Even countries long at odds with each other are sending humanitarian flights filled with needed medical supplies and ventilators. It is humbling and comforting to know that at our greatest time of need, we can come together.

But will the caring last? Will the social or physical distancing strategies have any long-term effects? Will there be renewed interest in the patient–provider relationship? Will documentation and regulatory requirements that deprive providers of face-to-face encounter time with patients be permanently waived? Will physical distancing remain a part of a healthcare visit? Will telehealth play a larger role in healthcare? Will hand sanitation and not touching your face remain a day-to-day priority?

My sincere hope is that part of this time's legacy will be that it restored humanity in healthcare. That caregivers of all types will have experienced renewal and place value on high-quality connections, empathetic listening, and emotional handling. That a profession once reduced to the perfunctory and routine will drive record numbers of students into healthcare who want to pursue such meaningful and impactful work. That respect, integrity, and high regard will return to the profession in overwhelming ways. That all of this will result in the enhancement of clinical outcomes by the combination of scientific evidence in medical interventions and the science of those transportable skills of positive psychology to the betterment of healthcare. That every day, each provider will remember something special—they were indeed Called to Care.

LARRY BENZ, SPRING 2020

What then is care? The word care finds its origin in the word kara, which means "to lament, to mourn, to participate in suffering, to share in pain." To care is to cry out with those who are ill, confused, lonely, isolated, and forgotten, and to recognize their pains in our own heart. To care is to enter into the world of those who are only touched by hostile hands, to listen attentively to those whose words are only heard by greedy ears, and to speak gently with those who are used to harsh orders and impatient requests. To care is to be present to those who suffer and to stay present even when nothing can be done to change their situation. To care is to be compassionate and so to form a community of people honestly facing the painful reality of our finite existence. To care is the most human gesture, in which the courageous confession of our common brokenness does not lead to paralysis but to community. When the humble confession of our basic human brokenness forms the ground from which all skillful healing comes forth, then cure can be welcomed not as a property to be claimed, but as a gift to be shared in gratitude.[1]

---

1   Nouwen, Henri J.M. *You Are the Beloved: Daily Meditations for Spiritual Living* (New York: Convergent Books, 2017), 193, Kindle.

INTRODUCTION

"The heart has its reasons which reason knows nothing of...We know the truth not only by the reason, but by the heart."

—BLAISE PASCAL

The above quotation has resonated with me throughout my adult life. It was the heart's reason that inspired me to become a physical therapist. I came to that decision when I was still very young, and I never wavered from it, even as I began to navigate the difficult path toward attaining a degree and credentials.

My first role as a physical therapist was treating soldiers. These were patients that placed their full faith in the practitioner's hands so they could diligently and quickly return to the field and fulfill their mission. The immediate feedback in terms of outcome and gratitude from these loyal soldiers enduring my early career in the US Army confirmed and solidified my decision to become a PT. As I entered the private practice world in the late 1980s, these same intrinsic motivators remained high for many years—until significant systemic changes began to derail the motivation of myself and others. These changes were the impetus for this book.

There have been two major occurrences in healthcare that, in my opinion, have had undesired effects for most providers. For many of us, these occurrences have reduced our calling to purposeful work and generated unprecedented levels of attrition, burnout, and disengagement. Over the past several years, in an attempt to make healthcare more efficient, various "process improvements" (excessive documentation, regulations, and a variety of other hoops and ladders) have replaced time spent with patients. External studies have documented that as much as 25 percent of a provider's time is not spent with a patient. Our internal studies show that for physical therapy encounters, the time spent away from patients is even greater. This time is now spent on unrelated but required administrative and insurance tasks that distract from provider-patient relationships and generally make healthcare worse for everybody.

The move toward and emphasis on evidence-based practice has also had another unintended and unfortunate consequence: providers now all too often focus excessively on techniques and proven interventions while overlooking cognitive or tacit knowledge skills—like how empathy, listening, communication, and collaboration can also affect healthcare outcomes. This unbalanced approach furthered my desire to put humanity back into healthcare and share what the research has to say about the so-called "soft" skills in medicine.

I have worked my entire career to make physical therapy a paradigm for innovative healthcare and have played various roles, including lobbying with colleagues to urge the passing of legislative changes in Kentucky, such as legislation bringing parity to physical therapy and primary care co-pays. This new legislation was a huge win for the physical therapy profession as it helped set a precedent for other states around the country where physical therapists were seeking similar change. I have also helped launch state and regional provider networks and coalitions whose mission is to improve business conditions for independent physical therapy practices nationwide.

My most recent years have been spent highlighting the cost-effectiveness and efficacy of "Physical Therapy First," which occurs when a patient accesses a physical therapist first for care after experiencing a musculoskeletal ache, pain, strain, or sprain and in particular if they have cervical or low back pain. When followed, patients benefit from faster recovery without drugs, imaging, or surgery, and employers and insurance companies benefit from resolved claims at significantly lower costs. Working with a variety of collaborators, this approach has proven out empirically in many markets across the US.

But throughout my career, I have been attracted to and intrigued by the nonclinical indicators of clinical success. For example, I have long wondered how a supervisor simply calling a work-injured patient within seventy-two hours of injury and telling him or her how much he or she has been missed might have a greater impact on whether this person comes back to work than various interventions, medications, and the passage of time. Or how is it that a subset of injured Army officers, upon learning that their x-ray results are normal, can have immediate and almost supernatural recoveries? Why did every one of my Haitian patients, following the 2010 earthquake, seemingly leave after treatment with a wide-eyed, so-called Duchenne smile despite my ability to offer only rudimentary interventions in substandard medical conditions? To the contrary, why do certain words and phrases inadvertently influence adverse effects or what is known as nocebo? We know that such nonclinical factors or what some call bedside manner are premier influencers of clinical outcome. The best current evidence refers to a more holistic "therapeutic alliance" and has garnered significant research interest.

My infatuation with this topic eventually led me to study the science of positive psychology via the University of

Pennsylvania's Master of Applied Positive Psychology Program (MAPP) where I soon discovered there was plenty of "reason" for these occurrences in the form of research. In 1998, Dr. Martin Seligman, incoming president of the American Psychological Association (APA), had challenged the field of psychology to broaden its focus to study and implement interventions that went beyond human problems and pathology to include the study of human strengths and well-being—basically, what's going right.[2] He thus initiated *positive psychology*, which is "a science of positive subjective experience, positive individual traits, and positive institutions."[3] Positive psychology takes a "strengths-based" approach to studying the specific ways people can build on their talents, skills, and values to generate greater happiness, success, and fulfillment. It is ripe with implications across a broad spectrum of professions, among them education, organizational scholarship, and healthcare.

Positive psychology literature has grown rapidly in significance since Seligman's challenge in 1998, generating over 18,000 scientific papers (2,300 were published in 2011 alone) and representing over 4 percent of *PsycINFO*,

2   Fowler, R.D., Seligman, M.E.P., and Koocher, G.P. "The APA 1998 Annual Report." *American Psychologist* 54, no. 8 (1999): 537-68. https://doi.org/10.1037/0003-066X.54.8.537.

3   Satterfield, J. M., "Happiness, Excellence, and Optimal Human Functioning: Review of a Special Issue of the American Psychologist, (2000;55:5-183), Martin E P Seligman and Mihaly Csikszentmihalyi, Guest Editors." *Western Journal of Medicine* 174, no. 1 (January 2001): 26-29. https://doi.org/10.1136/ewjm.174.1.26.

which is the largest source of psychological literature.[4] Still, there is little to no integration of its diverse topics within the healthcare profession, and the literature is even sparser in the field of physical therapy.

Most recently, I have been focused on integrating positive psychology into the clinical practice of physical therapy and healthcare in general. I began by going back to school and getting a master's degree in Applied Positive Psychology from the University of Pennsylvania. This program, under the direction of Dr. James Pawelski, was the first of its kind worldwide and was created by none other than Dr. Martin Seligman.[5]

In this era of enormous societal change, the pressure is now on healthcare executives to identify, adapt, and configure relevant healthcare technologies to yield greater efficiencies, reduce costs, manage greater transparencies, and cope with an environment now beset by rules, regulations, and insurance requirements. In 2014, the Physicians Foundation conducted a survey which received responses from 20,088 medical doctors and was reportedly the largest and most comprehensive survey of physicians as of that date.[6]

4   Rusk, Reuben D., and Waters, Lea E. "Tracing the Size, Reach, Impact, and Breadth of Positive Psychology." *The Journal of Positive Psychology* 8, no. 3 (2013): 207-21. https://doi.org/10.1080/1743 9760.2013.777766.

5   "Master of Applied Positive Psychology." The College of Liberal and Professional Studies (LPS), February 26, 2020. http://www.sas.upenn.edu/lps/graduate/mapp.

6   "2014 Survey of America's Physicians." The Physicians Foundation, n.d. https://physiciansfoundation.org/ focus-areas/2014-survey-of-americas-physicians-practice-patterns-and-perspectives/.

The survey contained some remarkable results:

- Over 51 percent of respondents were pessimistic about the future of healthcare
- 38.7 percent of respondents reported that medicine and healthcare were changing in such a way that they planned on accelerating their retirement plans
- 50.2 percent indicated they would not recommend the profession to their children
- 28.7 percent of respondents said they would choose a different career if they had to do it all over again
- Physicians noted that they were spending less time on patient care because paperwork was consuming 20 percent of their time
- Over 55 percent described their professional morale and feelings about the state of the medical profession as negative[7]

As a result of so many changes, *compassionate care* is all too often being replaced by *institutional care* characterized by electronic medical records (EMRs), coding, and algorithms. This is an unintended consequence of the focus on evidence-based practice, EMRs, and compliance, and it has resulted in provider burnout and patient dehumanization as demonstrated in the survey results. Provider burnout

7   "2014 Survey of America's Physicians." The Physicians Foundation, n.d. https://physiciansfoundation.org/ focus-areas/2014-survey-of-americas-physicians-practice-patterns-and-perspectives/.

impairs patient outcomes,[8] and dehumanization denies distinctively human concern for another human being[9]—particularly through the practice of depersonalization. First identified by the renowned psychoanalyst Isabel Menzies Lyth in 1960, depersonalization is manifested, in part, by the referencing of patients not by *name* but by *disease*.

My studies of positive psychology, combined with my experience in the real-life world of healthcare, ultimately led me to the initiative and formalized training program I have entitled Called to Care. Through its emphasis on relevant positive psychology concepts that we generally refer to as constructs (for example, leadership, kindness, compassion, and positivity), Called to Care has the opportunity to lead the effort in bringing humanity back into healthcare.

Through Called to Care, we hope to accomplish three primary objectives:

1. Promote and reinvigorate focus on compassionate clinical care
2. Renew call, purpose, and meaning for healthcare practitioners

---

8   Halbesleben, Jonathon R. B., and Rathert, Cheryl. "Linking Physician Burnout and Patient Outcomes." *Health Care Management Review* 33, no. 1 (2008): 29-39. https://doi.org/10.1097/01. hmr.0000304493.87898.72.

9   Haque, O.S., and Waytz, A. "Dehumanization in Medicine: Causes, Solutions, and Functions." *Perspectives on Psychological Science* 7, no. 2 (2012): 176-86.

3. Differentiate care and clinical outcomes for organizations adopting this training

Why should kind, compassionate, and positive care be such a point of emphasis? Evidence suggests that these things are greatly lacking—particularly with respect to listening and communicating. A Canadian and US study found that, on average, doctors interrupt patients within twenty-three seconds from the time a patient begins explaining his or her symptoms.[10] The same study found that during 25 percent of visits, doctors don't even ask patients what is bothering them. Another study that recorded thirty-four physicians during more than 300 patient visits found that doctors spent, on average, only 1.3 minutes conveying to patients crucial information about their conditions and treatment, and that most of the information doctors did provide was too technical for the average patient to grasp.[11] Interestingly, these same doctors estimated they spent more than eight minutes on this topic when asked.

Another study showed that three out of four doctors failed to give clear instructions to patients on how to take their

10   Marvel, M. Kim, Epstein, Ronald M., Flowers, Kristine, and Beckman, Howard B. "Soliciting the Patient's Agenda." *JAMA* 281, no. 3 (1999): 283-87. https://doi.org/10.1001/jama.281.3.283.

11   Stewart, M., Brown, J.B., Donner, A., McWhinney, I.R., Oates, J., Weston, W.W., and Jordan, J. "The Impact of Patient-Centered Care on Outcomes." *The Journal of Family Practice* 49 (2000): 796-804.

medicines.[12] And yet another study demonstrated that when asked to state their medication instructions, half of patients couldn't do it.[13] A 2011 Markle Foundation survey found that both patients and doctors agree that approximately 30 percent of the time, doctors forget important information that their patients tell them.[14] And finally, in a famous study on physician performance, patients received only 55 percent of the recommended care for thirty different medical conditions.[15]

These trends exist in many medical subgroups as well, including outpatient physical therapy. Our own internal studies show that more than 25 percent of a patient's encounter with us is spent on paperwork as opposed to direct patient care. To complicate the doctor–patient interaction, physical therapy has an additional concern: our patients typically have uninformed expectations in comparison to when they visit a primary physician.[16] Phys-

12   Vermeire, E., Hearnshaw, H., Van Royen, P., and Denekens, J. "Patient Adherence to Treatment: Three Decades of Research. A Comprehensive Review." *Journal of Clinical Pharmacy and Therapeutics* 26, no. 5 (2001): 331-42. https://doi.org/10.1046/j.1365-2710.2001.00363.x.

13   Brownlee, Shannon. "The Doctor Will See You–If You're Quick." *Newsweek*, April 15, 2012.

14   "Markle Survey: 70 Percent of Public Says Patients Should Get Summaries after Doctor Visits." Markle Foundation, January 2011. https://www.markle.org/publications/1442-70-percent-public-says-patients-should-get-summaries-after-doctor-visits.

15   McGlynn, E.A., Asch, S.M., Adams, J., Keesey, J., Hicks, J., DeCristofaro, A., and Kerr, E. "The Quality of Health Care Delivered to Adults in the United States." *The New England Journal of Medicine*, no. 348 (June 26, 2003): 2635-45. https://doi.org/10.1056/NEJMsa022615.

16   Roush, Susan E., and Sonstroem, Robert J. "Development of the Physical Therapy Outpatient Satisfaction Survey (PTOPS)." *Physical Therapy* 79, no. 2 (January 1999): 159-70. https://doi.org/10.1093/ptj/79.2.159.

ical therapy visits are also often longer and more frequent than most other medical visits, the diagnosis has typically already been settled, and the sessions require active participation from the patient that may be painful, which can be perceived as physically threatening.[17] All of this can cloud the effective delivery of compassionate care.

However, the lack of clear expectation also provides a significant opportunity for physical therapists to collaborate with patients, set realistic goals, and make joint decisions, which undoubtedly influence results. Engaging in a collaborative model of shared decision-making allows patients to feel in control of the healing process and their therapeutic decisions. A patient's autonomy increases ownership of the joint plan, enhances the therapeutic alliance between patient and doctor, and makes adherence to and engagement with the treatment more likely.[18]

The struggles that both healthcare providers and patients experience make healthcare an excellent industry for applying, developing, and refining evidence-based interventions and techniques from positive psychology. The alignment of these two disciplines presents a unique opportunity with the potential to substantially and positively impact

17   Linder-Pelz, Susie. "Toward a Theory of Patient Satisfaction." *Social Science & Medicine* 16, no. 5 (1982): 577–82. https://doi.org/10.1016/0277-9536(82)90311-2.

18   Data-Franco, J., and Berk, M. "The Nocebo Effect: A Clinician's Guide." *Australian and New Zealand Journal of Psychiatry* 47, no. 6 (2012): 1–7.

patient outcomes. Called to Care is a strategic initiative that translates relevant positive psychology concepts into clinical practice with the goal of better patient care.

We contend that there are three interrelated components to quality patient care experience:

1. *Clinical excellence*, or the degree in which the clinical skills, including critical thinking and integration of best evidence into treatment, contribute to a successful outcome.
2. *Service excellence*, which is exemplified by a defined and consistent approach to a customer service program. Our own program consists of ten principles that are taught, rewarded, emphasized, and monitored via third-party patient loyalty questionnaires, Net Promoter scores, and mystery shoppers.
3. *Care and Compassion excellence*, the very subject matter of this book cultivated through a Called to Care initiative. This includes a myriad of clinician and patient interactions and interventions along with practitioner reflections and experiences.

These three interrelated components must have distinct, systematic initiatives in order to be fully integrated within any particular practice. It was determined that a strategic plan for Called to Care must consist of *experiential, collaborative, didactic,* and *monitoring* mechanisms in order to comprehensively persuade healthcare practitioners to integrate it into their practices and sustain the change. The developed plan consisted of the recruitment of willing physical therapists, an orientation via an introductory video, and a half-day Appreciative Inquiry (AI) Summit followed by a self-paced, online learning management teaching and facilitation.

To test the efficacy of Called to Care, 1,314 physical therapy patients evaluated the behaviors of forty Called to Care-trained physical therapists via the Consultation and Relational Empathy (CARE) Measure, a validated instrument that assesses key clinical experiences like empathy, listening, and positivity. The results, when compared to a normative database of physiotherapists who did not receive training, showed significant findings. Patients truly have enhanced experiences when their therapists receive specialized training in these areas. And, as a result of our work, we are also convinced that we have far too much data, too many regulations, and too many constraints in healthcare—and not enough care. If you are reading this book, I am sure you agree.

The result of all this is a course that is designed to rehumanize healthcare by:

- Correlating clinical outcomes with empathy, compassion, high-quality connections, placebo/nocebo

research, and portable concepts within the field of positive psychology
- Helping healthcare practitioners find renewed purpose, meaning, and calling in their careers, which also reduces provider burnout and attrition
- Engaging in the power of Appreciative Inquiry (AI) to strengthen and heighten the positive potential between healthcare practitioners and patients

This book is the culmination of my work, which also involved my comrades within the physical therapy profession who willingly embraced excellence in care and compassion and whom I know to be "Called to Care." This book shows how to integrate the most relevant evidence-based positive psychology topics and interventions into modern-day healthcare practices. *Called to Care* utilizes the science of positive psychology to train healthcare practitioners to enhance important behaviors like listening, empathy, and positivity, facilitate better patient experiences that influence clinical results, renew or enhance each healthcare practitioner's sense of purpose, and provide differentiation—far different than what today's patients have unfortunately come to expect.

In November 2013 when I received the Robert G. Dicus Award, the most highly regarded award in private practice physical therapy by our professional association, I shared the implications of positive psychology with several thousand of my colleagues. During my acceptance speech, I asked them to look beyond a patient's physical recovery and consider the importance of interventions that enhance overall well-being. My experience with healthcare providers of all types is that they, too, are called to purposeful and meaningful work. This book enables us to start deploying the *Called to Care* platform to healthcare practitioners across the United States and abroad, integrating it into their entry-level training, and elevating the experiences of patients and healthcare practitioners alike. My hope is that this book allows all healthcare providers to know the truth—through reason, but especially in their hearts.

How This Book Is Organized

Each chapter represents a construct, technique, or intervention that Called to Care providers incorporate into their caregiving. At the end of each chapter, you will find a list of available resources and tools that encourage, support, provide excellent examples, and provide references and evidence for their support. A skill checklist is also included at the end to serve as a handy reference and reminder to incorporate these skills into daily practice. All of these are also available at CalledtoCaretheBook.com.

CHAPTER ONE

HIGH-QUALITY CONNECTIONS AND EMPATHY

PUTTING "CARE" BACK INTO HEALTHCARE

"Seeing with the eyes of another, listening with the ears of another, and feeling with the heart of another."

—ALFRED ADLER

Jane, an experienced physical therapist, is listening intently to the components of empathy during an academic lecture entitled "Emotional Handling," the idea of acknowledging a patient's feelings or simply asking about how they feel about something. The realization that empathy has essentially four components has her surprised. The instructor elaborates, "The second kind of empathy, affective empathy, is less about the cognitive ability to understand where a person is coming from than about sharing or mirroring another person's emotions. So, if I see my daughter crying in anguish and I too feel anguish, then I am experiencing affective empathy as I feel the emotion and legitimatize it. If, on the other hand, I notice her anguish but feel a different emotion, such as pity—*oh, the poor little thing,* I might think— then I am showing sympathy rather than empathy. Sympathy typically refers to an emotional response that is not shared." Even more striking is the instructor's reflective question: "Would your opinion and treatment of the patient change if you admitted you didn't know everything about them?"

Jane reflects on her years in patient care. She remembers the times when patients told her something about their amount and location of pain that didn't align with Jane's knowledge of anatomy and physiology. She could have accepted and recognized her patient's emotions and perspectives, seeing it as their truth rather than disregarding it as irrelevant and choosing to skip over the conversation and onto the more comfortable area for Jane—the physical exam. This reflection is heartfelt—she knows she wasn't providing the most impactful care and she was imposing her thoughts and judgments. She vows to be empathetic in its full dimension and to not simply go into a default mode of sympathy, exam routine, and problem-solving.

What a High-Quality Connection Feels Like between Practitioner and Patient

The award-winning 2001 film *Wit* depicts the struggle of Vivian Bearing, a scholar of John Donne's poetry of irony who is dying from ovarian cancer.[19] In one of the final scenes, her mentor comes to visit. Shocked at the suffering of her former student, the graduate-school professor doesn't try to console Vivian with words but simply crawls into bed with her and reads to her from a children's book about enduring and unconditional love. According to Johanna Shapiro and Lloyd Rucker, many medical students are moved to tears by this scene, and subsequent discussions enable students as well as medical providers to move from the level of concrete reality to that of idealism.[20] As these medical students further reflect, they are moved to report feeling not only empathy but also sorrow, care, and compassion. They admire the experience behind the old professor's spontaneous gesture; furthermore, the image of Vivian Bearing, dying and embraced, becomes fixed in these soon-to-be physicians' minds as a representation of all they want to realize in their treatment of their future patients.

From a healthcare perspective, empathy is the ability to

---

19 *Wit*, directed by M. Nichols (2001; United States: Home Box Office Films).

20 Shapiro, Johanna, and Rucker, Lloyd. "The Don Quixote Effect: Why Going to the Movies Can Help Develop Empathy and Altruism in Medical Students and Residents." *Families, Systems, & Health* 22, no. 4 (2004): 445–52. https://doi.org/10.1037/1091-7527.22.4.445.

put yourself in another person's shoes without judgment. That means you envision things from that person's perspective, attempt to feel what he or she is feeling, and behave in a supportive manner. For countless reasons, empathy has all too often become a lost art in healthcare. However, the industry may also simply be reflecting society at large, which has become increasingly complex, pressured, and competitive.

In our daily practices, we can begin restoring empathy in healthcare by building on a foundation of mutual positive regard, trust, and active engagement—things that are at the core of a high-quality connection.

The best healthcare professionals establish high-quality connections with their patients so that they can discuss the patients' expressed needs, concerns, and emotions, as well as discern their patients' unexpressed needs, concerns, and emotions. They do this by:

1. Incorporating *emotional handling*, making sure to ask about feelings and acknowledging and legitimizing the patient's emotions.
2. *Empathetic listening* or the assurance of really being *other*-centered by the perspective of yourself in another person's shoes—intellectually and emotionally.
3. Mindfulness (further explored in chapter 10), which

repels a natural inclination to be influenced by first impressions or diagnosis bias.

4. An attitude of humility, which allows the practitioner to work in collaboration with the patient (versus from a position of power). It has been demonstrated that power positions actually decrease the ability of mirror neurons to resonate or be in sync, which in turn reduces empathy.

As Jane realized while listening to the lecture, a high-quality connection starts with an admission and a realization that we don't know all we need to know about another person; therefore, it is our job to listen and learn as much as we can by actively attending to all the cues conveyed by the patient's words and actions, and then act accordingly. Far too often, healthcare providers get the action component of empathy but intervene without engaging the other key components of empathy. But high-quality connections are all about being genuine, communicating affirmation, effective listening, and supporting a comfortable communication style.

Connection quality is marked by three subjective experiences:

1. It is sensed by feelings of strong, active energy known as vitality. People in a high-quality connection are more

likely to feel positive arousal and a heightened sense of positive energy.[21]

2. The quality of a connection is felt through a sense of positive regard.[22] Being regarded in a positive context means you experience feelings of being loved, respected, and cared for in a connection.[23] Positive context in the face of healthcare concerns, which are predominantly negative, might appear contradictory, but that is what makes a Called to Care practitioner differentiating—these practitioners have the ability to be personally enriching, genuine, and positive in environments that are difficult.

3. It is marked by the degree of shared feeling known as mutuality. Simply put, it is the sense of this being a high-quality connection. Shared mutuality captures the bidirectional vulnerability and responsiveness that both people feel when they are fully engaged in a connection.[24]

These three subjective markers—vitality, positive regard, and mutuality—help explain why high-quality connections

21 Quinn, Ryan W., and Dutton, Jane E. "Coordination as Energy-in-Conversation." *Academy of Management Review* 30, no. 1 (2005): 36-57. https://doi.org/10.5465/amr.2005.15281422.

22 Rogers, C.R. *Client-Centered Therapy: Its Current Practice, Implications and Theory.* Boston, MA: Houghton Mifflin, 1951.

23 Stephens, J.P., Heaphy, E., and Dutton, J. *The Oxford Handbook of Positive Organizational Scholarship.* Edited by Kim S. Cameron and Gretchen M. Spreitzer. Oxford; New York: Oxford University Press, 2013.

24 Miller, Jean Baker, and Stiver, Irene Pierce. *The Healing Connection: How Women Form Relationships in Therapy and in Life.* Boston, MA: Beacon Press, 1998.

are experienced as attractive and pleasant and why they are not only life-giving but actually make patients feel more cared for and lead to more successful outcomes.[25]

We must never forget the words of William James, the father of American psychology, who once said that "the deepest principle in human nature is the craving to be appreciated." This is the reason why high-quality connections are vital to the energy of any organization. In my experience, most patients as healthcare consumers have never been told they are appreciated—we have forgotten they are the most important characters in the healthcare arena. Thus, the empirical evidence on the psychological, physiological, and behavioral benefits of high-quality connections are core to the teachings of *Called to Care*.

How Exquisite Empathy Is Also Good for Practitioners

In a 2009 study, researchers wanted to find out why successful mental health professionals were able to sustain long-term careers with little burnout. Mental health professionals generally have the highest rate of burnout versus anyone else in healthcare, and the hypothesis going into the study was that clinical detachment would

25 Stephens, J.P., Heaphy, E., and Dutton, J. *The Oxford Handbook of Positive Organizational Scholarship*. Edited by Kim S. Cameron and Gretchen M. Spreitzer. Oxford; New York: Oxford University Press, 2013.

mean less burnout. Interestingly, this research found just the opposite: those *most* engaged with their patients had the *lowest* levels of stress.[26] The researchers found that mental health professionals who exhibited *exquisite empathy*—defined as being highly present, sensitively attuned, and well-boundaried while creating heartfelt empathetic engagement—were invigorated versus depleted by intimate professional connections with traumatized patients. This protected the practitioners against compassion fatigue and burnout.

Physicians and therapists who make more time for caring and learn to love even their most difficult patients can potentially become better caregivers with more successful medical outcomes. They also happen to be happier people.

Unfortunately, these days, the medical system often encourages professionals to *unlearn* empathy by shifting the practitioner's attention to compliance, documentation, productivity demands, and superimposed rules and regulations. Further exacerbating this problem is that many young people are now unlearning whatever empathy skills they developed growing up in a culture that focuses more on social media status than cooperation and values.

---

26 Harrison, Richard L., and Westwood, Marvin J. "Preventing Vicarious Traumatization of Mental Health Therapists: Identifying Protective Practices." *Psychotherapy: Theory, Research, Practice, Training* 46, no. 2 (2009): 203-19. https://doi.org/10.1037/a0016081.

Is there hope for those of us who might be suffering from a lack of empathy? Can we regain this all-important skill?

Becoming Better at Empathy Can Be as Simple as Watching a Movie

In the 2004 study involving the movie *Wit*, researchers Johanna Shapiro and Lloyd Rucker confirmed the importance of the humanities and arts in enhancing empathy. They called the acquisition of empathy through watching movies and reading literature the "Don Quixote Effect." Don Quixote is the seventeenth-century story of a Spanish landowner who reads romantic tales about knights and princesses. Emulating his imaginary heroes, he suits up in makeshift armor—accompanied by his faithful, yet skeptical, squire Sancho Panza—and sets out to accomplish deeds of daring and gallantry. He battles windmills that he fantasizes to be giants, chases sheep he thinks are armies, and idolizes a common peasant woman as though she were a princess. His delusions enable him to find meaning, beauty, and love in life.

Sadly, the extreme nature of Don Quixote's idealism causes all who cross his path to react with scorn as his "Quixotic" dreams often cause harm to others. However, the pragmatist, Sancho Panza, who knows that none of this is real, ends up exemplifying chivalry through loyal, courteous, and protective love. The knight and squire ironically end up becoming a lot more like each other as they both are simultaneously admiring and critical of their heroic quests. Thus, it is not Don Quixote who is the role model for medical students. The lesson comes in his "Don Quixote Effect" on his practical servant, Sancho, who allows himself, on occasion, to live in Don Quixote's world and become a more honorable and tender person. Through this story, we as practitioners can be inspired to be more in the world of our patients, just as the medical students who watch *Wit* were inspired to become more caring.

Shapiro and Rucker's study is not the only to demonstrate this effect. Lancaster, Hart, and Gardiner (2002) offered a one-month course for medical students in which the students read stories such as Leo Tolstoy's *The Death of Ivan Ilyich*. In the evaluation at the end of the course, students assigned their highest rating to the enhancement of their empathy.[27] Similarly, researchers Shapiro, Morrison, and Boker (2004) noticed a significant improvement in first-year medical students' empathy after they participated in a short course in which they read and discussed poetry, skits, and short stories.[28] Ultimately, the students understood

---

27   Lancaster, Tim, Hart, Ruth, and Gardner, Selena. "Literature and Medicine: Evaluating a Special Study Module Using the Nominal Group Technique." *Medical Education* 36, no. 11 (2002): 1071-76. https://doi.org/10.1046/j.1365-2923.2002.01325.x.

28   Shapiro, Johanna, Morrison, Elizabeth, and Boker, John. "Teaching Empathy to First Year Medical Students: Evaluation of an Elective Literature and Medicine Course." *Education for Health: Change in Learning & Practice* 17, no. 1 (January 2004): 73-84. https://doi.org/10.1080/1357628031 0001656196.

that it was their attention to humanities that facilitated their behavioral change.

All of this supports the use of arts, namely literature and film, to build up the empathy muscle—a key recommendation for the Called to Care practitioner. Such movies as *The Fisher King* (Gilliam and LaGravenese, 1991), *Terms of Endearment* (Brooks and Brooks, 2005), *The Philadelphia Story* (Demme and Nyswanger, 1993), and, of course, *Wit* (Nichols, Thompson, and Nichols, 2001) should be a routine part of the healthcare practitioner's arsenal. Literature has likewise been shown to benefit an increase in tolerance for uncertainty and an enhanced grounding for empathic understanding of patients.[29] Of course, we are seeking similar results through the Called to Care initiative.

For a deeper dive into empathy, go to the presentation on "10 Things Health Care Practitioners Need to Know about Empathy" at CalledtoCarethebook.com.

Clinical Case: Empathy in Action

Jose was a young physical therapist who had a deep desire to work with complex musculoskeletal patients—those who often presented themselves with obesity, low back pain, type 2 diabetes, and deconditioning. He was drawn to this

---

29   Hojat, M. "Ten Approaches for Enhancing Empathy in Health and Human Services Cultures." *Journal of Health and Human Services Administration* 31, no. 4 (2009): 427.

population because of his upbringing in a predominately Hispanic community in San Antonio that had been ravaged by these and other healthcare problems. His patient, Maria, fit the prototype well.

Earlier in his career, Jose would typically get a brief history, pinpointing the issues to address and then immediately go into "I'm a PT mode" by lining out a treatment plan as opposed to really connecting with the patient. Jose had always graded himself high in empathy because of his call to action for this affected population—but not any longer, once he learned that prosocial concern was just one construct of empathy. Since that realization, Jose has applied a different strategy that takes into account a high-quality connection through an energized approach of positivity and vitality. He decided to listen attentively in a positive, shared connection.

While truly listening to Maria's plight, Jose was able to access shared experiences and mutuality as he distinctly recalled with great emotions the trials and tribulations of his own aunt, who had a remarkably similar history to Maria. Instead of going through the motions of pretending, or what some would call surface acting, with Maria while already lining out a treatment plan, Jose instead took the harder path of going deep and really seeing Maria's perspectives while not judging her alcohol abuse, obesity, and bad eating habits. In turn, Jose was able to recount to Maria his own experience with his aunt, and the two became incredibly connected in a highly engaged and emotionally charged conversation.

This flowed into the physical exam and a conversation on goal setting. Adding further value, Jose used an evidence-based technique that enhances compliance in diabetics—the use of a best-self exercise, one in which Maria envisions herself already healthy and flourishing. Then, and only then, and in collaboration with Maria, did the last component of physical therapy intervention, and the one most likely aligned with prosocial concern ensue: treatment planning consisting of graded exercise prescription, manual therapy, and pain neuroscience education. Jose's practice of empathy is highlighted by better care and higher odds of the best clinical outcome, a highly engaged patient, and his own meaning of purposeful work to which he was called years ago.

For more resources on this topic, visit CalledtoCarebook. com.

CHAPTER TWO

BROADEN-AND-BUILD

THE SCIENCE OF POSITIVITY

"The psychological broadening sparked by one positive emotion can increase an individual's receptiveness to subsequent pleasant or meaningful events, increasing the odds that the individual will find positive meaning in these subsequent events and experience additional positive emotions."

—BARBARA FREDRICKSON

When you walk into a medical office in the United States these days, you're typically met with paperwork clipped neatly onto a board with a pen and a chain, which is something akin in today's world to Flintstones medicine. You know the paperwork will ask you, in a million different ways, what's wrong with you. You ask about the amount of paperwork and are told in so many words that the regulations, insurance companies, and federal government require it along with so many of your signatures. So, you take a deep breath and find a leather chair. You look around the room and are met with forlorn faces tucked into magazines. However, it's clear those faces aren't really focused on the news, gossip, or lifestyle advice found in those pages; they're waiting to be needled, probed, queried, and hurried so they can hear what's wrong with them, get fixed, and be sent on their way. But what if a visit to the doctor could look completely different than that?

In advance of your visit to a Called to Care physical therapy clinic, you are sent a personalized email with an option of filling out the paperwork in advance, along with a link to an app that gives you the ability to interact with a real person from the start, including to do online scheduling. A short video tells you about your personal physical therapist and care team, as well as the experience you will have on the first visit. When you arrive for your first visit, you are greeted warmly by a friendly and compassionate front desk worker—referred to as a care coordinator—who makes you feel comfortable and affirms you are in the right place at the right time. Very quickly afterward, you have used an iPad to self-report on a survey that facilitates your recovery and your personal physical therapist escorts you to a room where, perhaps for the first time ever, someone listens to you for quite a while before they even examine you.

Regardless of whether we are working in physical therapy or another modality, how can we make positive health-care experiences more the norm for everyone involved? Fortunately, a renowned researcher, backed by plenty of replication, has provided us with some direction.

The Broaden-and-Build Theory of Positive Emotions

Barbara Fredrickson's broaden-and-build theory of positive emotions illuminates the importance of positivity for broadening our mindsets and expanding our range of vision and possibility.[30] Broaden-and-build theory clarifies the science behind why high-quality connections promote openness, knowledge, exploration, innovation, and solutions to problems, and it is this science that medical providers must embrace and implement.

The theory might be best understood by first considering the opposing mindset: *stress*. When we become stressed, we tend to become narrow-minded and undergo a myriad of negative physiological challenges like higher blood pressure, a quickening pulse, and spikes in cortisol. We're mentally prepared

---

30 Fredrickson, Barbara L. "The Role of Positive Emotions in Positive Psychology: The Broaden-and-Build Theory of Positive Emotions." *American Psychologist* 56, no. 3 (2001): 218-26. https://doi.org/10.1037/0003-066x.56.3.218.

for "fight" or "flight"—or, given our present-day realities, to hit *send* on that email. In his 1996 book, *Emotional Intelligence: Why It Can Matter More than IQ*, Daniel Goleman used the term "amygdala hijack" to describe such emotional responses, which are often immediate, overwhelming, out of measure with the current stimulus, and often on par with a much more significant threat.[31] While this phenomenon is more complex and nuanced than what was traditionally believed to be happening, there is no question we can likely all think of a time in our lives when "fire, aim, ready" was our response to a trigger or stimulus. Medical providers who are stressed through regulatory requirements and productivity workplace demands are not immune to this scenario.

Fredrickson's broaden-and-build theory of positive emotions is part of Called to Care because of its potential benefits to patients, healthcare practitioners, and workplace dynamics. The theory says that positive emotions broaden thought and action, enabling individuals to be flexible in higher-level connections and consider wider-than-usual ranges of precepts, ideas, and actions. Very often, the formality of a healthcare environment contributes a sharp contrast to what a "broaden-and-build" mindset purports, thus the necessity for frequent reminders of the impact of positive emotions regardless of setting. The broaden-and-build theory of positive emotions says

31 Goleman, D. *Emotional Intelligence: Why It Can Matter More than IQ.* New York: Bloomsbury Publishing, 1996.

that a broadened thought process enhances flexibility that, in turn and over time, builds personal resource availability, including mindfulness, resilience, social closeness, and even physical health.[32,33,34] As such, it is best thought of as a gift that keeps on giving.

Fredrickson likens the effect of positivity to the heliotropic effect of plants when they turn toward the light, reaching open to take in as much as possible. Positivity and open-mindedness are freed and feed upon each other, creating upward spirals of positivity. Positive thoughts lead to more expansive, creative decision-making, improve the ability to find solutions to problems, and create more trusting relationships.

Broaden-and-Build in the Digital Era

As an example, let's consider a problem that many of us know all too well these days: information overload. Every medical environment has direct access to a variety of internet-enabled technologies. While this digital era allows

---

32 Cohn, Michael A., Fredrickson, Barbara L., Brown, Stephanie L., Mikels, Joseph A., and Conway, Anne M. "Happiness Unpacked: Positive Emotions Increase Life Satisfaction by Building Resilience." *Emotion* 9, no. 3 (2009): 361-68. https://doi.org/10.1037/a0015952.

33 Fredrickson, Barbara L., Cohn, Michael A., Coffey, Kimberly A., Pek, Jolynn, and Finkel, Sandra M. "Open Hearts Build Lives: Positive Emotions, Induced through Loving-Kindness Meditation, Build Consequential Personal Resources." *Journal of Personality and Social Psychology* 95, no. 5 (2008): 1045-62. https://doi.org/10.1037/a0013262.

34 Waugh, Christian E., and Fredrickson, Barbara L. "Nice to Know You: Positive Emotions, Self-Other Overlap, and Complex Understanding in the Formation of a New Relationship." *The Journal of Positive Psychology* 1, no. 2 (2006): 93-106. https://doi.org/10.1080/17439760500510569.

us to access information used in patient care and to see a much bigger picture about our organizations, lives, and relationships, it's gotten all too easy to get bogged down by compulsions to surf, to access social media, and to look at news, online ratings, and reviews. Depending on the day, you may find this avalanche of information to be enlightening, daunting, or overwhelming. Regardless, it's happening. And the higher up you are in your organization, the more you will be impacted by the intrusions of these modern-day "efficiencies." Thus, it's important to develop new strategies to move our organizations forward in this era, utilizing new data and technologies as tools to fuel broader, more realistic, and richer views of our organizations and lives, so they can be contributing factors rather than distracting. The new strategy of broaden-and-build can be adopted and developed and can significantly impact personal relationships at a time when our digital distractions de-emphasize and monopolize our relationship time.

Broaden-and-build, when adopted by healthcare practitioners and utilized in patient care interactions, also provides lasting and enhanced benefits that transport outside of the patient care setting. This is because inducing positive emotions increases people's ability to be in community or close with others[35] and also increases their trust

---

35 Waugh, Christian E., and Fredrickson, Barbara L. "Nice to Know You: Positive Emotions, Self-Other Overlap, and Complex Understanding in the Formation of a New Relationship." *The Journal of Positive Psychology* 1, no. 2 (2006): 93-106. https://doi.org/10.1080/17439760500510569.

in acquaintances.[36] Thus, extending broaden-and-build to the practitioner's life outside of healthcare elevates benefits to many others.

As theorized, broaden-and-build's impact is in combining what is referred to as hedonic well-being, or the experience of pleasant emotions with eudemonic well-being, or the striving toward your potential and purpose in life. The benefits of this impact are that it brings about an accumulation of skills and resources one can leverage in one's relationships, most notably the heightened sensitivity around the role that social and emotional factors play on our thoughts and behaviors.[37] This newly developed skill, often referred to as a component of emotional intelligence, has significant implications for our patients. Even though the pleasant, positive emotions that we use in our interactions with them may seem fleeting, they actually have a longer-lasting effect on the patient and improve functional outcomes that, in turn, lead to greater well-being and connectedness. In this way, our use of positive emotions expands other people's

---

36 Dunn, Jennifer R., and Schweitzer, Maurice E. "Feeling and Believing: The Influence of Emotion on Trust." *Journal of Personality and Social Psychology* 88, no. 5 (2005): 736-48. https://doi.org/10.1037/0022-3514.88.5.736.

37 Kashdan, Todd B., Biswas-Diener, Robert, and King, Laura A. "Reconsidering Happiness: The Costs of Distinguishing between Hedonics and Eudaimonia." *The Journal of Positive Psychology* 3, no. 4 (2008): 219-33. https://doi.org/10.1080/17439760802303044.

mindsets and curiosity in ways that, little by little, can reshape their lives.[38]

We can extend this to our organizations and patients. The practice of medicine is infiltrated with formality in a mostly insulated environment through language, dress, rituals, reams of paperwork, waiting rooms, clinician mannerisms, and often hard-to-understand terminology that has to be interpreted by the patient as positive or negative.[39] This all imparts significant meaning to patients. This meaning then influences patients' emotions and, thus, their outcomes.[40] So let's look more closely at how all the small choices we make and deciding to be focused on helpful words and techniques every day can have a huge impact on our patients and their outcomes.

Health Implications of Positivity for Our Patients

Placebo research has taught us that the simple use of a sugar pill can have dramatic clinical effects. Borrowing from this and relative evidence, we know that healthcare

---

38   Garland, Eric L., Fredrickson, Barbara, Kring, Ann M., Johnson, David P., Meyer, Piper S., and Penn, David L. "Upward Spirals of Positive Emotions Counter Downward Spirals of Negativity: Insights from the Broaden-and-Build Theory and Affective Neuroscience on the Treatment of Emotion Dysfunctions and Deficits in Psychopathology." *Clinical Psychology Review* 30, no. 7 (2010): 849–64. https://doi.org/10.1016/j.cpr.2010.03.002.

39   Swindell, J. S., Mcguire, A. L., and Halpern, S. D. "Beneficent Persuasion: Techniques and Ethical Guidelines to Improve Patients' Decisions." *The Annals of Family Medicine* 8, no. 3 (January 2010): 260–64. https://doi.org/10.1370/afm.1118.

40   Swindell, J.S., Mcguire, Amy L., and Halpern, S. D. "Shaping Patients' Decisions." *Chest* 139, no. 2 (2011): 424–29. https://doi.org/10.1378/chest.10-0605.

professionals influence their patients by how they communicate—specifically choosing enabling words over those that trigger. For example, normative aging findings on x-ray can be called "arthritis" or "wrinkles on the inside" but the former can lead a patient to believe they have something seriously wrong while the latter may guide them to believe they are aging normally.

Therapeutic alliance refers to the relationship between a healthcare professional and a patient. It is the means by which a provider and patient hope to engage with each other and affect beneficial change in the patient. Methods for enhancing this alliance include setting mutually agreed expectations, discussing relative treatment approaches underpinned with scientific evidence that the patient can understand, and creating a more relaxed and natural setting. This nurturing increases perceived ownership of the shared plan and makes adherence and engagement with treatment more likely. This alliance is the key supportive relationship that is the hallmark of what is referred to as patient-centered care.

Healthcare professionals would benefit from a detailed study on specific methods that enhance meaningful effects via positivity, problem framing, patient engagement, and the use of ritual; these therapeutic adjuncts should prioritize a patient's preferences to optimize positive outcomes. Here is a short list of examples:

1. Person-first communication versus defining by disability: "Mr. Jones" versus "the knee patient"
2. Providing affirmation: "I am here to be as helpful as possible."
3. Establishing a connection that enables rapport: "What is your preferred name that I should use?"
4. Personalized instruction: "What is your preferred method of learning this exercise—a picture or video, I demonstrate, or you perform and I provide instructions as you are doing it?"
5. Personalized follow-up: "Do you prefer a reminder call, text, or email?"

Not surprisingly, it is not just the interactions between the provider and patient that matter but the total exposure to the experience, including reception, scheduling, and billing and collections departments. Inadvertent word choices can influence, imprint, and impact a patient just as profoundly as their provider.

Colleagues of mine at the International Spine and Pain Institute have culled the research and developed an online course entitled "Words that Harm and Words that Heal in the Front Office"[41] which has become a mandatory part of our training. This online class, using the latest neuroscience research, provides attendees with an understanding

---

41   "Words that Harm and Words that Heal in the Front Office." Evidence in Motion. Accessed June 2, 2020. http://evidenceinmotion.com/wthh.

of how pain works and showcases current front-office and medical interactions that can harm patients, sometimes unknowingly. On the flip side, the presentation features various front-office strategies that can help patients along their recovery path, starting with the first phone call. Medical care starts and ends in the front office, and for too long, this important factor has been overlooked.

As further evidence has evolved, it points to multiple body systems that positivity impacts. Fredrickson and Levenson have shown that positive emotions, both amusement and contentment, can speed up cardiovascular recovery from anxiety and fear. Perhaps even more significant, positive emotions have been shown to help patients rebound from adversity, cardiovascular reactivity, ward off depressive symptoms, and continue to grow.[42,43,44]

42 Fredrickson, Barbara L., Tugade, Michele M., Waugh, Christian E., and Larkin, Gregory R. "What Good Are Positive Emotions in Crisis? A Prospective Study of Resilience and Emotions Following the Terrorist Attacks on the United States on September 11th, 2001." *Journal of Personality and Social Psychology* 84, no. 2 (2003): 365-76. https://doi.org/10.1037/0022-3514.84.2.365.

43 Ong, Anthony D., Bergeman, C. S., Bisconti, Toni L., and Wallace, Kimberly A. "Psychological Resilience, Positive Emotions, and Successful Adaptation to Stress in Later Life." *Journal of Personality and Social Psychology* 91, no. 4 (2006): 730-49. https://doi.org/10.1037/0022-3514.91.4.730.

44 Tugade, Michele M., and Fredrickson, Barbara L. "Resilient Individuals Use Positive Emotions to Bounce Back from Negative Emotional Experiences." *Journal of Personality and Social Psychology* 86, no. 2 (2004): 320-33. https://doi.org/10.1037/0022-3514.86.2.320.

The Positivity Ratio

So, how much is enough? Can we ever have too much of a good thing?

Barbara Fredrickson's research looked to answer this question. She undertook this research with a Chilean psychologist by the name of Marcial Losada. Together, they looked at interactions in corporate settings to determine the typical ratio of positive to negative words used in everyday exchanges. It turns out that flourishing teams have a 2.9- or, really, a three-to-one ratio of positive statements to negative statements in their meetings and interactions. Stagnating teams have a much lower ratio, and bankrupt companies have ratios far below that.[45] Fredrickson and Losada (2005) suggest that a person's overall affect and general well-being are represented by his or her "positivity ratio," defined as the ratio of positive to negative emotions experienced over time.[46] Normal functioning has been characterized by a positivity ratio of about two-to-one.[47]

But patients may have medical conditions that could subject

45 Bakker, Arnold B., and Schaufeli, Wilmar B. "Positive Organizational Behavior: Engaged Employees in Flourishing Organizations." *Journal of Organizational Behavior* 29, no. 2 (2008): 147-54. https://doi.org/10.1002/job.515.

46 Fredrickson, Barbara L., and Losada, Marcial F. "Positive Affect and the Complex Dynamics of Human Flourishing." *American Psychologist* 60, no. 7 (2005): 678-86. https://doi.org/10.1037/0003-066x.60.7.678.

47 Schwartz, Robert M., Reynolds III, Charles F., Thase, Michael E., Frank, Ellen, Fasiczka, Amy L., and Haaga, David A. F. "Optimal and Normal Affect Balance in Psychotherapy of Major Depression: Evaluation of the Balanced States of Mind Model." *Behavioural and Cognitive Psychotherapy* 30, no. 4 (2002): 439-50. https://doi.org/10.1017/s1352465802004058.

them to negativity biases. For example, negative emotions, events, and problems may command attention and prevent individuals from assessing situations evenhandedly.[48] This suggests that in order to overcome the potency of negative emotions, positive emotions must outnumber them by more than two-to-one (i.e., normal functioning). Losada and Heaphy (2004) identified the three-to-one ratio as a key ratio; above this ratio, optimal functioning emerges.[49] This was further tested by Fredrickson and Losada (2005), who found that when people are above the three-to-one ratio, they experience the broaden-and-build effects of positive emotions and went on to demonstrate cooperation with peers and family, personal growth, and the ability to rebound. When the ratio dips below three-to-one, positivity did not move the needle in terms of having any measurable effect.[50] Thus, a three-to-one (or greater) ratio should exist with your patients, in your interactions with your coworkers, and in your personal life if you want all these areas to flourish. Although there have been recent challenges to some specifics of the three-to-one calculation by Losada in terms of whether it can really be defined by such a numerical formula, the consensus remains that a ratio in this range

48 Rozin, Paul, and Royzman, Edward B. "Negativity Bias, Negativity Dominance, and Contagion." *Personality and Social Psychology Review* 5, no. 4 (2001): 296–320. https://doi.org/10.1207/s15327957pspr0504_2.

49 Losada, Marcial, and Heaphy, Emily. "The Role of Positivity and Connectivity in the Performance of Business Teams: A Nonlinear Dynamics Model." *American Behavioral Scientist* 47, no. 6 (2004): 740–65. https://doi.org/10.1177/0002764203260208.

50 Keyes, Corey L. M. "The Mental Health Continuum: From Languishing to Flourishing in Life." *Journal of Health and Social Behavior* 43, no. 2 (2002): 207. https://doi.org/10.2307/3090197.

is necessary, and you have to have significantly greater positive (versus negative) interactions.

You've learned about the broaden-and-build theory, and how achieving a certain ratio of positive-to-negative thinking can help you, your coworkers, and your patients. It blends emotions with purpose, brings skills and resources, including emotional intelligence, and results in connectivity, curiosity, and enhanced well-being.

Our organization views positivity as a competitive advantage in the marketplace because it is teachable, energizing, and enables flourishing. This, in turn, leads to better clinical outcomes, a richer and more pleasing environment to work in, and better, kinder, more compassionate patient care. The application of positive psychology in modern-day medicine is becoming clear. Positivity is a learned skill that pays off not only in your own life but also in the lives of everyone who comes into contact with you. This is the perfect antidote for what is ailing us in healthcare. This is the essence of *Called to Care*.

For more resources on this topic, visit CalledtoCarebook.com.

CHAPTER THREE

SELF-EFFICACY

THE VITAL SIGNIFICANCE OF CONNECTIONS

"I think I can, I think I can."

—*THE LITTLE ENGINE THAT COULD*

One of my favorite patients ever was Tommy, a Green Beret who suffered from multiple lower extremity trauma injuries after a parachute jump on a windy day. His desire and motivation were inspiring, his understanding of rehab concepts uncanny, and his attendance 100 percent. We were preparing to get him back in marching shape, which for a Green Beret typically means covering ten-miles-plus of ground while wearing a thirty-pound or more backpack. All of Tommy's physical measurements lined up, and I assured him that he was ready and that we should simply start with a few hundred yards.

After fifty feet, Tommy sat down and would not continue. This fear-avoidance phenomenon is common and cannot simply be cured by cajoling or encouragement. Working through this takes empathy and a high-quality, trusting connection over a period of time. I asked Tommy about his career marches—the ones that went well and the ones that didn't and, in particular, what he was feeling with each. We talked openly about fear and anxiety as well as making sure it was understood that from a physical standpoint, there wasn't anything we were going to do that would trigger or cause more damage to his healed injuries. Tommy had done marches for years in his storied career, and he acknowledged that his physical capacity at this stage of his rehab was adequate for what I asked him to do. The issue was Tommy simply didn't believe he could do it.

For the next few sessions, we focused on a pact and a phrase we co-created: "believing is seeing." For military personnel, pacts or agreements are binding commitments that reinforce duty, honor, and loyalty. Applying this to recovery is a simple but effective concept. Tommy would repeat my belief in him as his PT, "Tommy, your body says it can achieve." He would then leverage the confidence I had in him with a gain in confidence in himself. He learned through the repeated sessions that his prior pain and discomfort from his injuries were gone and that, in fact, increasing activity had no impact on his pain, nor did it cause reinjury. We introduced breathing exercises that are known to calm anxiety. Visual imagery, or the focused attention of seeing himself marching in his own mind, was adapted between sessions and initiated with every session. He began to see himself marching just as proficiently as when he was a younger soldier. As this process evolved over a few days, turning into a few weeks, Tommy easily marched the minimal distance and then independently worked out and eventually completed all the physical demands, including the lengthy marches required for his Green Beret status. They say "seeing is believing," but more often, and in particular, in healthcare, belief comes first and "believing is seeing" is a far more effective mantra.

Understanding the Power of Nurturing Self-Efficacy

Even when you're having a bad day, it's vitally important to focus on and listen to your patients and optimize your time with them. This may sometimes mean that you have to force yourself to forget about everything else around you—even the ringing phones and patients in the waiting room—in order to better engage with the patient directly in front of you. As we saw in our story about Jose, once you have a high-quality connection, your patient will trust you more, and trust becomes the currency of mutual relationships that enables patients to open up about their spoken and unspoken needs. You can then utilize the mutuality of the relationship to tap into and enhance your patient's *self-efficacy*, that is the belief in his or her abilities to produce desired results through his or her own actions. For example, a patient who trusts you is more apt to listen to your advice on changes to his or her diet and exercise and will be more likely to comply with your recommendations.

This type of interaction is the foundation of self-efficacy, which is one of the most important aspects of facilitating recovery. In fact, self-efficacy may be the most important factor in physical rehabilitation. Additionally, self-efficacy has been found to be a strong factor associated with less pain-related disability among older veterans with chronic pain. Research has also shown that greater self-efficacy is also associated with higher levels of exercise adherence in healthy populations as well as compliance and long-term exercise adherence for those undergoing cardiac rehabilitation.

Other studies have assessed self-efficacy and its role in patient adherence to physical therapy or in any kind of recovery in terms of performing home exercise and engaging in long-term prevention strategies. Tijou, Yardley, Sedikides, and Bizo (2010) found that self-efficacy and the degree in which patients understood outcome expectancies predicted attendance and performance in actual physical therapy and via completion of the prescribed number of sessions they were instructed to attend.[51] In other studies,

---

51 Tijou, Imogen, Yardley, Lucy, Sedikides, Constantine, and Bizo, Lewis. "Understanding Adherence to Physiotherapy: Findings from an Experimental Simulation and an Observational Clinical Study." *Psychology & Health* 25, no. 2 (2010): 231–47. https://doi.org/10.1080/08870440802372431.

Cressman and Dawson found self-efficacy was enhanced by the use of imagery or the ability for a patient to visualize their success, which led to a higher likelihood of completion of physical therapy exercises and satisfaction with rehabilitation.[52]

Where We Get Our Sense of Self-Efficacy From

Again, self-efficacy refers to people's beliefs in their own capabilities to produce the desired effects through their own actions. A strong sense of self-efficacy has many benefits, including improved physical health and well-being. A weak sense of self-efficacy can have negative consequences, such as depression, anxiety, and avoidance behavior.

To get a better sense of the concept, reflect back on a daunting activity in your past, like diving off the high board for the first time when you were a child. This was likely to have been frightening at first, and that fear may have even caused you to refrain from even trying. However, if you watched your friend attempt the dive without fear, this may have emboldened you. That's because our sense of self-efficacy is enhanced or diminished as we integrate experiences, information, and feedback from different sources:

52 Cressman, Joel M., and Kimberley A. Dawson. "Evaluation of the Use of Healing Imagery in Athletic Injury Rehabilitation." *Journal of Imagery Research in Sport and Physical Activity* 6, no. 1 (2011): 1–24. https://www.semanticscholar.org/paper/Evaluation-of-the-Use-of-Healing-Imagery-in-Injury-Cressman-Dawson/0762ba7d37ff22ba702776ba7588a4c5db6d fbc4.

- *Our performance experiences*: the amount of success we attribute to our own efforts in a given scenario
- *Our vicarious experiences*: our observation of others engaging in a behavior, particularly if they are perceived as being similar to us
- *Verbal persuasion*: the influence of a trusted source
- *Our physiological and emotional states*: these are particularly significant when success is associated with positive feeling states.[53]

Healthcare practitioners have the opportunity to build a patient's self-efficacy. Here is a short checklist that has strong evidentiary support:

1. Through verbal encouragement, not just passively watching. "Joe, your form and pace were right on!"
2. Facilitating positive feeling states. This includes the use of specific language that resonates with the patient, which can vary greatly from patient to patient. "Mary, just think of how much fun you and your husband, Joe, will have going back to your walking routine."
3. Highlighting and capitalizing on the patient's progress. This includes reminding the patient where they were at in prior sessions and how far they have progressed.
4. Sharing success stories associated with similar patients.

---

53   Maddux, J.E. "Self-Efficacy: The Power of Believing You Can." In *Oxford Handbook of Positive Psychology*, edited by S.J. Lopez and C.R. Snyder, 2nd ed., 335-43. New York: Oxford University Press, Inc., 2009.

For patients undergoing rehab post total hip and knee replacements, spine surgery, and shoulder surgery, we provide with permission a patient ambassador of similar demographics who has agreed to be a reference and speak to their rehab and recovery.

To further optimize a patient's self-efficacy, healthcare practitioners should be prepared to give up a certain amount of status or control in order to empower their patients. All too often, the focus has been on us as providers from a position of authority. Our agenda, if not checked, can project an image of some supernatural power to fix our patients rather than as an educator and an enabler. By changing our mindset from one of control to one of support and service, we aid greatly in the healing process as well as develop a relationship based on mutuality. The oft-served phrase "Get over yourself" is applicable here. Patients are best served when we are viewed as equals. As we learned in chapter 2, the mere act of a humble, supportive countenance creates greater resonance, which neurologic research says enhances mirror neurons and, therefore, empathy. It's not the practitioner as a power broker, but the healthcare provider as an equal to the patient that leads to success. So, sit down with your patient, be transparent, fully display your own humanness and the result will be mutuality, which will elevate your patient's self-efficacy.

The Relationship between Self-Efficacy and Proxy Efficacy

One final concept to add to self-efficacy is more about you than your patient. At least, at first it is. Proxy efficacy is our confidence in the skills and abilities of a third party (or parties) to function effectively on our behalf. For the sake of our discussions, it is your patient's belief in how great you are.

An interesting study on self-efficacy by Bray and Cowan (2004) assessed the relationship between self-efficacy and confidence in practitioners.[54] Patients participated in a highly structured and individualized biweekly exercise program; data were captured for five months. The researchers utilized a developed scale for exercise self-efficacy and a modified scale for the assessment of proxy efficacy. Results generally supported the hypotheses, meaning the results showed proxy efficacy to be a potent variable that predicted exercise self-efficacy, attendance, and post-program exercise intentions. The evidence strongly suggests that medical practitioners should encourage self-efficacy and use motivational interaction because they are likely to improve attendance, enhance compliance, and foster better clinical outcomes.

Don't we all want our patients to have confidence in us?

---

54   Bray, Steven R., and Cowan, Heather. "Proxy Efficacy: Implications for Self-Efficacy and Exercise Intentions in Cardiac Rehabilitation." *Rehabilitation Psychology* 49, no. 1 (2004): 71-75. https://doi. org/10.1037/0090-5550.49.1.71.

Of course, we do—and it's not because of ego. We've seen in physical therapy that when patients possess strong proxy efficacy, they have great confidence in their providers, adhere to their exercise programs (during and after formal programs), and, most importantly, attend their sessions. When our patients believe in us, they experience better outcomes.

Interestingly, the research shows that *self-efficacy* equals *proxy efficacy*. The more that people believe in themselves, the more they will believe in you. This is very similar to Charles Horton Cooley's 1902 social psychological concept, the looking-glass self, which essentially states that our sense of self is an outgrowth of our interactions with others; thus, our own sense of worth is connected to how others engage and interact with us.

You can get your patients to believe more in themselves with positive instructions and motivational interactions. Traditionally, providers simply enter rooms and start with procedures like blood pressure, respiration, and pulse rate. Contrast this norm with a simple way that is not only more courteous but also encourages self-efficacy—asking for permission before you do something. For example, you might say:

"Could you please put this medical gown on?"

"Do you mind if I enter the exam room?"

"Is it OK with you if I take your blood pressure?"

It is easy to forget that patients come to us for help and deserve respectful service. Organizations all over have responded to this notion by adopting or developing customer service systems within the healthcare environment. This trend has gained momentum, and key hospital systems are attempting to differentiate based purely on a customer service focus. Likewise, we have for many years taught a proprietary program called AmaZing!, which patient satisfaction and loyalty surveys have empirically supported. These systems, while important, do not serve as a substitute for care and compassion initiatives like Called to Care, which access critical psychological interventions and concepts like self-efficacy, positive emotion, and high-quality connections, and significantly influence clinical success.

These concepts all clarify a final important thought. Can you remember a time when a challenging patient with low self-efficacy had a physiological or psychological effect on your well-being? How did this affect your communication, positive engagement, and motivation?

It's clear that our sense of purpose as healthcare providers influences our patients' levels of satisfaction, which then tends to influence our satisfaction as providers. This is why the lessons in *Called to Care* are so important. Strategies for compassionate, kind, and positive care help change outcomes and enhance the self-efficacy of our patients. The use of high-quality connections, broaden-and-build, and positivity all result in enhanced outcomes because of this belief called self-efficacy.

Maddux summarizes three decades of research showing that our sense of self-efficacy is the most important thing in determining what we choose to do, how long we persevere at it, and how far we succeed. "When equipped with an unshakeable belief in one's ideas, goals, and capacity for achievement," he explained, "there are few limits to what one can accomplish."[55] This is the sense of positivity and confidence we need to cultivate in our patients.

For more resources on this topic, visit CalledtoCarebook. com.

---

55   Maddux, J.E. "Self-Efficacy: The Power of Believing You Can." In *Oxford Handbook of Positive Psychology*, edited by S.J. Lopez and C.R. Snyder, 2nd ed., 335-43. New York: Oxford University Press, Inc., 2009.

CHAPTER FOUR

THE ART AND SCIENCE OF POSITIVE INTERACTIONS

ACTIVE CONSTRUCTIVE RESPONDING

"There is no bad time for good news."

—STEPHEN KING

Imagine an after-dinner scene at a long-term care facility in Florida. A few dozen residents have gathered to play games, talk, watch television, and visit with family members. Suddenly, the peaceful scene is shattered when an eighty-nine-year-old man falls out of his wheelchair. In short order, staff members rush to assist, have him transported to the nearest hospital, and contact his children.

Over the next five days, the man makes only modest progress. His head and right arm sustained serious injuries. Chances of a full recovery are slim. However, on the sixth day, he comes out of his haze, eats a few bites of ice cream, and says a few words. This marks the beginning of a return to health. Hospital personnel share the exciting news with his children, who travel to the hospital from their disparate locations and gather around their father. More milestones quickly ensue.

Two days later, the man returns to the long-term care facility. Upon arrival, staff members ask detailed questions about his time at the hospital. Upon hearing about his initial achievements, they follow up with positive comments like, "That must have felt great! Can you tell me more?" Healthcare specialists pick up this line of questioning as well as the attendant enthusiasm the next day.

I'm sure I don't even need to point out that this particular man had excellent social support in his life. In the context of our discussion, "social support" can include the social connections that a person reports, specific support given, and perceived support, like the perception that others will come to your aid if needed.[56] Research indicates that perceived support is consistently associated with positive health and well-being.[57] When someone tells their friends and loved ones that they will be there for them during tough and troubling times, this support and care validate the relationship, reduce anxiety and depression, and result in a positive experience.

As such, the social support that a healthcare provider extends through their mere transparency, availability, and communication readiness imparts a significant benefit to the provider-patient relationship and assists in patient recovery. While privacy laws and technology can be constraints, Called to Care providers find means through applications and telehealth to communicate their support and availability. But there is even a more profound method.

The Importance of Capitalization and Active Constructive Responses

Capitalization is defined as the process of informing another person about the occurrence of a personal, posi-

---

56 Gable, Shelly L., and Gosnell, Courtney L. "The Positive Side of Close Relationships." *Designing Positive Psychology: Taking Stock and Moving Forward*, 2011, 265-79. https://doi.org/10.1093/acprof: oso/9780195373585.003.0017.

57 Kaul, Manju, and Lakey, Brian. "Where Is the Support in Perceived Support? The Role of Generic Relationship Satisfaction and Enacted Support in Perceived Support's Relation to Low Distress." *Journal of Social and Clinical Psychology* 22, no. 1 (2003): 59-78. https://doi.org/10.1521/jscp.22.1.59.22761.

tive event and thereby deriving additional benefit from it.[58] You tell someone about something good that happened to you, and you get to enjoy it all over again. In effect, a person recounting a positive experience gets additional bang for the buck or receives additional enhancement beyond the benefits associated with the positive event itself. When implemented properly, capitalization fosters:

1. Reliving and reexperiencing the event
2. Rehearsal and elaboration, which enhances the experience
3. Memory access: you remember events that you communicate about frequently.
4. Positive social interactions: you are perceived positively in the eyes of others, thus enhancing connection with others (validating and caring).

But as healthcare practitioners, we have to be careful when a patient relates good news to us. It is very easy for us to accidentally quash their enthusiasm and miss an opportunity to have them capitalize on their success. Thankfully, it is also very easy to encourage them. Let's say, for instance, that a patient reports positive news to you. She tells you that since her last appointment, she went for a mile-long

58   Langston, Christopher A. "Capitalizing on and Coping with Daily-Life Events: Expressive Responses to Positive Events." *Journal of Personality and Social Psychology* 67, no. 6 (1994): 1112–25. https://doi.org/10.1037/0022-3514.67.6.1112.

walk with her spouse. You have four ways that you could, in theory, respond to this good news:

1. *"Great! That has got to make you feel super! Tell me about the walk; was it in your neighborhood?"* This would be something known as active constructive responding or enthusiastic support.
2. *"That's great! Let's go ahead and get this physical therapy session started."* This is passive constructive or quiet, understated support.
3. *"Oh my, be careful! That's progress, but you might not be able to do that next time—especially with the type of injury you have."* This is known as active destruction or simply quashing an event.
4. In this case, you just totally ignore your patient and move on to a new activity in a new session. This is known as passive destructive.

According to well-documented studies by Shelly Gable and her colleagues, only active construction positively correlates with commitment, satisfaction, intimacy, trust, and relationship quality while all others negatively correlated with these measures.[59] When you passively construct, and by the way, just using single words like "nice," "great," and "cool" are considered passive, you not only fail to help the

59 Gable, Shelly L., Reis, Harry T., Impett, Emily A., and Asher, Evan R. "What Do You Do When Things Go Right? The Intrapersonal and Interpersonal Benefits of Sharing Positive Events." *Journal of Personality and Social Psychology* 87, no. 2 (2004): 228–45. https://doi.org/10.1037/0022-3514.87.2.228.

patient capitalize but you also decrease commitment, satisfaction, intimacy, trust, and the quality of the relationship because you have not really engaged with the patient in a resonant way.

Gable et al. (2004) studied active constructive responding (ACR) extensively, including studies with couples, and have found that positive-event discussions—and thus ACR—were more closely related to current relationship commitment, satisfaction, love, well-being, and a diminished risk of breaking up down the line. Interestingly, the relative importance of the event for men did not matter; they want all positive events to have enthusiastic support. For women, the capitalization response by their partner to events that they deem important was crucial.

Within the context of a clinical visit, on days when people communicated their positive events to others, they experienced greater positive affect and satisfaction with life, above and beyond the importance of the event itself. The beauty of positive emotions, broaden-and-build, and the use of self-efficacy facilitation and active constructive communication is that they all create an upward spiral that gives patients that connection they need to experience tremendous benefits that they credit to their clinical experience and what happens to them when they leave the healthcare environment. Perhaps more importantly, the patient's clinical improvement is facilitated, and patients are comfortable returning to this environment if a new or recurrent problem occurs as well as when they recount to their family, friends, and coworkers their overall experience with the clinic and the practitioner. Said differently, a patient in painful rehabilitation for a shoulder injury shows improvement in their range of motion, strength, and function, along with a positive affect and experience that lasts far outside of their time in the physical therapy clinic. A patient undergoing care for their cardiovascular diagnosis receives benefits through these nonclinical techniques and interventions far exceeding improvement to their heart. Both patients tell their circles of family, friends, and colleagues.

Be Ready to Be Active

In healthcare, there are endless opportunities to respond to patients' good news. For example, in nursing and primary care, patients talk about their accomplishments in terms of their psychological well-being, mood, affect, and sleep quality. In rehabilitation settings, patients often talk about their physical accomplishments, like walks, lifting abilities, work, exercises, improved ability to work a few hours, and even the ability to sit up and watch a movie.

Nevertheless, as a PT, I unfortunately remember many times when I responded to a patient's good news with something like, *"Good, glad to hear it. Now let's get on with our session and get to work."* This failure to capitalize meant a failure for the patient to experience the intrinsic goodness of the event an additional time.

So that you are ready...here are a few phrases to keep in your repertoire that actively construct and enhance your relationship, drive commitment, and trust:

"Wow! That's incredible! Tell me about it!"

"That had to make you feel wonderful today!"

"That's fantastic! How did that make you feel?"

"I am so proud of your accomplishment! How do you feel about it?"

"Your hard work and diligence is paying off! What do you think?"

It's Part of Your Job to Facilitate Capitalization

Called to Care healthcare practitioners, take mindful advantage of capitalization opportunities whenever possible by not just listening to a patient recount their positive experience, but facilitating them to share it and experience it a second time. Patients, in this way, are actively participating in their own recovery, which switches their relationship with their healthcare provider from one of dependence to one of equals. In this respect, the provider that takes advantage of capitalization is not mindlessly defaulting to the role of "fixer" in the relationship, but a mutual environment is assured, and further progress is enabled.

So, the next time you hear, "Oh, I'm so excited! I was able to walk an additional fifty feet today!" you might consider responding, "Wow! That's incredible! Tell me about it! That had to make you feel wonderful today!"

For more resources on this topic, visit CalledtoCarebook. com.

CHAPTER FIVE

GOAL SETTING

AN RX FOR POSITIVE CHANGE

"The great secret about goals and visions is not the future they describe but the change in the present they engender."

—DAVID ALLEN

Jane resides at an assisted living facility. After being independent, she spent several weeks in inpatient rehab following a series of small strokes. Her providers at every setting, from acute care to her current facility, provided her with care that was focused on her physical stature and function—from the strength of her arms to her ability to walk independently. While she progressed, something was missing and her current occupational therapist, Jody, noticed it immediately—the goals were always to get well enough to graduate to the next setting, from initial stages in the hospital to skilled care, inpatient rehab, and now home health in an assisted living facility. In short, Jane had been cared for not based on her goals and aspirations but by the external financial incentives that drive patients to the least costly setting of care. So-called care pathways have created milestones that permit discharging patients based on clinical criteria that enables a facility to make more money by decreasing lengths of stay by receiving a bulk payment regardless of how much time or care is required for the patient.

Jody, being an astute Called to Care therapist, immediately tried to help Jane into a new narrative after six weeks of treatment that was focused on the payment of her multiple strokes, not on her goals and desires. Jody immediately prioritized learning goals that would enable Jane to demonstrate proper self-care and management with adaptive equipment. She instituted performance goals on objective measures of progress in ambulation and strength, including the ability for Jane to hold her great-grandchild. Lastly, a key intrinsic goal was crafted based on Jane's ultimate dream—to be active with her great-grandchild at her neighborhood playground.

Goal Setting

Goal setting is essential when we seek to undertake any large tasks in our lives—whether it be writing a book, starting a business, changing long-term habits, losing weight, or recovering from an illness. We often find the most potential for attaining our goals and creating change by working toward our goals steadily, consistently, and over time instead of trying to accomplish such tasks all at once or seemingly overnight. For example, when I wrote this book, I worked on a certain number of pages at a time and over a couple of years instead of trying to complete the entire manuscript in a month or two. Thus, we can use our ability to break things down and to set appropriate goals to attain our larger goals in life.

As we work with patients on setting realistic and positive goals, we need to show them how they can actively participate in generating better health outcomes for themselves. This process should help our patients to focus their attention on variables under their control, recognize and celebrate incremental improvements, and realize more positive outcomes. Even with terminal illnesses such as Alzheimer's, goal setting can provide a roadmap to mitigate certain symptoms, slow progression, optimize quality of life, and increase opportunities for attaining desired outcomes.

While there may be compliance and reimbursement rules and regulations associated with certain goals in healthcare, we must work to ensure that they do not interfere with more insightful patient-stated goals. In fact, we should strive to maintain a focus on letting our patients tell their stories, which are elicited through high-quality connections, empathy, positivity, and active constructive communication. Patients can have a best-imagined future self if we just remember to ask them.

To increase our effectiveness with our patients when it comes to the goal-setting process, we can start by familiarizing ourselves with a few well-researched types of goals that are particularly relevant for patient care and relate to each other: *performance goals, learning goals*, and *intrinsic goals*.

The Three Types of Goals You'll Need to Understand

A *performance goal* is the typical one we focus on in rehabilitation. This is any goal that involves measurable performance and enables patients to have at least some control over associated outcomes. For best results, performance goals should always be challenging and highly specific. For example, you might say to a friend that you are going to start running a certain number of miles a day, are planning to double this by the end of the summer, and are aiming to run a certain number of miles in a certain timeframe by autumn.

Learning goals are also effectively utilized in healthcare settings, such as rehabilitation; they involve setting specific outcomes, which provide context for predicting performance. For example, the goals set by Jody for Jane to demonstrate proper self-care with adaptive equipment. In our chronic pain patients, we set learning goals of mindful breathing techniques to deal with potential pain triggers that can mitigate the deleterious effects of stress. There is a promising trend of dieticians emphasizing learning goals these days. For example, some will take their patients grocery shopping and teach them how to become more proactive in maintaining their health through nutrition and proper food choices. In our experience, learning goals are still all too often ignored in healthcare where the most common default is to prioritize the requirements of insurance companies over patient-centered care. This is unfortunate because many patients are motivated and driven by learning and often seek us out specifically for prevention, information, and skills rather than just applied interventions.

An *intrinsic goal* is a goal set by a patient and not by anybody else like family, friends, culture, or teammates. They are based exclusively to the personal interest of the patient. For this reason, intrinsic goals can inspire passion and commitment, can produce outcomes that are more satisfying and meaningful, and may even induce states of flow. "Flow" is the feeling we get when we are lost in time because the task at hand is matched to meeting a challenge. Contrast an intrinsic goal to an extrinsic goal, one that is focused on outside validation including aspirations of fame, money, or beauty. In healthcare, external regulatory agencies compel providers to set goals that meet stringent requirements or risk not being a covered service. It is then incumbent upon the provider to demonstrate that those goals are being addressed in the care of the patient—for example, a total knee patient requires a certain range of motion, strength, and walking distance. This is far different than that same total knee patient stating that their personal goal is to be able to walk in the park with their mate. Facilitating these intrinsic goals is an essential skill of a Called to Care practitioner.

The secret sauce of developing intrinsic goals is to ask questions in a process known as patient inquiry. For example, you might ask your patients:

- How will you benefit from this goal that you are setting for yourself?
- What will it take for you to achieve this goal?
- How will achieving this goal make you feel?
- Why is this goal important to you?
- How will your life be better?

This facilitation is necessary because patients traditionally are not asked about their own goals and desires. In our experience, new providers are often taken aback by the suggestion that the patients can be empowered to make their own goals explicit. The typical physical and occupational therapy note, as well as Medicare's requirements, mandate the use of "short- and long-term goals" that are written in a very medicalized fashion. Our suggestion is to always include a section regarding patient aspirations or goals from their treatment sessions. Combining this with very specific performance and learning goals can ensure a patient-centered plan to success.

Start Goal Setting for the Future

Another key to helping your patients with goal setting is to understand the *contrasting effect*. To effectively utilize this technique, you begin a goal-setting process by establishing your patient's vision of an ideal future self and contrasting this with his or her current condition. For example, your patient's vision of parenthood versus their current state of obesity-related infertility. This enables you to create motivation, optimism, and positivity within your patient. In this situation, a patient might be more receptive to making significant lifestyle changes—finding a less stressful job, losing weight, and actively working to build a happier and healthier lifestyle—in order to attain his or her dream of becoming a parent.

The focus on best future vision is in sharp distinction from the traditional goal-setting model where the current condition is the point of emphasis and is compared to where the patient wants to be after treatment. The traditional model is not nearly as effective or engaging for the patient. Therefore, as you work with your patients, always try to start with the end in mind rather than current state by co-creating a picture of the patient's ideal future self and then work backward to optimize the patient's chances for success. All too often, we simply default to the matter at hand. But it is best to start with the best future self—not where the patient is at right now. Pair this with performance, learning, and intrinsic type of goals, and a successful outcome will be optimized.

Example: Barbara had just received a total joint surgery and is now at home receiving nursing and physical therapy, having had the surgery performed in an outpatient surgical center. Traditional goal-setting conversation explains or demonstrates to Barbara about her current state, the range of motion in her hip and knee, her ability to transfer from the bed to sitting and standing, and the number of steps she can currently make with the assistance of her walker. This current status is then projected on a goal. "Our goal is to get you from lying to sitting, to standing, to walking one hundred feet with your walker." In the contrasting goal-setting technique, the caregiver asks the patient to envision her best future self. Barbara glows as she details what she envisions: playing golf with her Thursday afternoon group, afternoon strolls with her husband, and driving the grandchildren around. The caregiver can then set the goals by working backward, all the while emphasizing Barbara's best ideal self, post hip surgery.

Choose the Hard Goals—Because They're Hard

Additionally, it also turns out that hard goals—not soft or easy ones—are the way to go. Hard goals require a longer commitment, greater attention, and more diligence. For our patient Jane, it was more about carrying her great-grandchild rather than just holding her at the playground. People who are optimistic about achieving their goals but expect it to be hard succeed far more often than people who are only focused on their current ideal futures. Findings from multiple studies on aspirational or "hard" goals show that the pursuit of goals outside of a person's comfort zone resulted in greater feelings of authentic self-esteem at the end of the day.

The evidence is convincing. Regardless of whether one is a student, worker, or patient, clear-cut goals are a recipe to flourish. For this reason, Called to Care therapists use the evidence of goal setting to maximize outcomes on all levels with their patients.

Goal Setting in Action

Let's now pull all of this together. Imagine a middle-aged man who is currently taking blood pressure medication. He would prefer not to take medicine if he doesn't have to. During a routine physical exam, he shares this with a nurse practitioner (NP). The NP begins with some inquiry about the patient's ideal future self. She finds out that he feels he is too young to be on the medicine, doesn't like the thought of being on it for the rest of his life, and wants to make lifestyle changes to attain his best future goal of getting off all medication. The NP comes up with the idea of setting lifestyle goals like eating a healthier diet by first understanding what type of diet he should be on (learning goal), consuming less salt (hard goal), and increasing cardiovascular exercise (performance goal) as these may help manage blood pressure in some situations.

The patient agrees to commit to these lifestyle changes (hard goals) and sees the NP again in three months. At this stage, they agree to take him off the blood pressure medication as long as the patient can continue to work on his lifestyle goals. He does and visits the NP again in another three months. His blood pressure is completely fine. Thus, in this scenario, the patient's goal of getting off blood pressure medication could be achieved by establishing healthy lifestyle goals.

When you begin with the ideal future (in this case, getting off blood pressure medication) and compare it to present-day conditions (i.e., contrasting thinking), you create motivation, optimism, and positivity toward making it happen. As you now understand, contrasting thinking isn't quite as successful if you start with where the patient is now and compare this with where he wants to be. You have to start with the ideal future as envisioned by a conversation and an image—established by you and the patient—and then work backward.

Goals = Conversation

Did you notice that throughout this chapter there was a common theme? That theme was that all this goal setting was occurring within the context of a *conversation* with the patient. These conversations are occurring all the time in healthcare, and your patients' goals should be revamped as often as necessary. After all, we are not setting goals for our patients; it is our work to extract the goals that are most important to them and then use our expertise to support them in succeeding.

Mastering the art of goal setting can be of enormous benefit; therefore, it is highly advisable to utilize the research associated with goal setting to maximize outcomes with your patients. It is part of the entire arsenal of *Called to Care*, transporting the research of positive psychology to healthcare.

For more resources on this topic, visit CalledtoCarebook. com.

CHAPTER SIX

THE SCIENCE BEHIND THE PLACEBO RESPONSE

"The placebo effect is the single greatest indicator that your capacity to heal starts in your mind."

—AUTHOR UNKNOWN

Dr. Tackett is a home health therapist working with Bill, a middle-aged, knee replacement patient. Bill has been experiencing a lot of pain, which is not uncommon at this stage of his rehab and has unfortunately kept him from doing his range of motion and strengthening exercises. His lack of progress has led him to a second knee manipulation—a procedure whereby under anesthesia, his knee is manually forced to achieve a further range.

Dr. Tackett decides to dig deep to not only treat the physical issues the patient is having but to also connect at a deeper level, including explanations of the source and influences of our fear and anxiety around pain. Bill is placed in an immersive virtual reality environment via VR goggles with some breathing, visualization, and illustrations. Bill's expectations about getting pain-free and back to being mobile are enhanced by providing positive information about the treatment and plenty of reassurance by Dr. Tackett and the VR narrations. A huge influencer to Bill is the now-solidified understanding that most patients have a pain barrier to overcome and, through encouragement, successfully go on to more difficult exercises and interventions.

As an added piece, Dr. Tackett joins the patient directly in the exercises, and Bill noticeably has better tolerance. At the next and future visits, Bill is much more compliant and has actually done some of the exercises on his own at home, aiding greatly to his own recovery. Bill and his personal physical therapist, Dr. Tackett, celebrate this achievement, proceed with treatment again, and the patient is significantly happier and gaining in progress.

The Physical Power of Placebo

A few years ago, I co-authored an article and subsequent responses with Dr. Timothy W. Flynn for the *Journal of Orthopaedic & Sports Physical Therapy.*[60] The article explored how placebo and nocebo phenomena can affect the relationship between the physical therapist and patient to the point that patient outcomes may be considerably influenced. This article, "Placebo, Nocebo, and Expectations: Leveraging Positive Outcomes," cited research over the past decade that has allowed a traditional understanding of placebo and nocebo effects (as a psychological response) to shift to that of a real, psychobiological response.

But what exactly are placebo and nocebo effects?

- "Placebo" means "I shall please" in Latin. In the case of placebo, a patient's symptoms may improve while he or she is receiving an inactive substance in a clinical trial.
- "Nocebo" means "I shall harm" in Latin. In the case of a nocebo, a patient experiences adverse or harmful effects while receiving an inactive substance.

Studies show that positive expectations—like our home health therapist telling the knee replacement patient that other patients tolerate the treatment well—are foretelling of favorable treatment outcomes. Conversely, low expectations foretell undesirable outcomes. The behavior of practitioners carries heavy weight in both scenarios, and

60 Benz, Laurence N., and Flynn, Timothy W. "Placebo, Nocebo, and Expectations: Leveraging Positive Outcomes." *Journal of Orthopaedic & Sports Physical Therapy* 43, no. 7 (2013): 439-41. https://doi.org/10.2519/jospt.2013.0105.

the knowledge that these phenomena strongly affect the relationship between patient expectations and outcomes has obvious and powerful consequences within the physical therapy profession and many facets of healthcare, in general. In our article, we argued that the combination of evidence-based interventions and the framing of experiences in a positive manner by therapists can radically change patient encounters.

We, as part of Called to Care, should obviously try as much as possible to embrace placebo while trying to negate nocebo and thus attempt to positively influence outcomes. Furthermore, we should think of these effects as nonspecific. *Specific* effects are what your intervention is intended to do based on your judgment, experience, and the evidence for it. Specific effects are caused by the elements of the intervention. Nocebo and placebo fall into nonspecifics—but that does not mean they should not be considered when it comes to your behavior and treatment choices.

This past decade has provided a rich and nuanced understanding of the placebo effect, and we now know that placebo and nocebo are real psychobiological responses to healthcare interactions.[61] However, there remains a gross misperception about placebo. Even medical practitioners

---

61 Sanderson, Christine, Hardy, Janet, Spruyt, Odette, and Currow, David C. "Placebo and Nocebo Effects in Randomized Controlled Trials: The Implications for Research and Practice." *Journal of Pain and Symptom Management* 46, no. 5 (2013): 722–30. https://doi.org/10.1016/j.jpainsymman.2012.12.005.

think that placebo is a mental or psychiatric phenomenon. The truth is that there has been a ton of research that clearly demonstrates a measured biologic response. For example, it has been shown that naloxone (a drug that reverses an opioid overdose) blocks a placebo pain-relieving response; the response is mediated by neural pathways involved in pain and opioid responses.[62] Additionally, functional magnetic resonance imaging demonstrates activity within various parts of the brain, brainstem, and spinal cord during a placebo-demonstrated, pain-relieving response.[63] Thus, the research supports that placebo is indeed biologic or physical. Certainly, there is a mental component to it; however, it is not a mental-only response.

How to Effectively Use Placebo in Your Practice

One way to enhance the placebo effect is through positive communications. Your ability to communicate with your patients in a positive way will influence outcomes. In fact, there have been over twenty-five randomized control trials that have found that demonstrated improvements, or what are known as "enhancing patterns," result from positivity.

---

62 Lieberman, Matthew D., Jarcho, Johanna M., Berman, Steve, Naliboff, Bruce D., Suyenobu, Brandall Y., Mandelkern, Mark, and Mayer, Emeran A. "The Neural Correlates of Placebo Effects: A Disruption Account." *NeuroImage* 22, no. 1 (2004): 447–55. https://doi.org/10.1016/j.neuroimage.2004.01.037.

63 Oken, B. S. "Placebo Effects: Clinical Aspects and Neurobiology." *Brain* 131, no. 11 (2008): 2812–23. https://doi.org/10.1093/brain/awn116.

When we provide the support of reassurance, we support and affect health outcomes in a positive way.

For example, there was a study that involved 200 patients who had symptoms, but no abnormal findings, and they also had no diagnoses that could be made.[64] They were randomly assigned to a treatment or no-treatment group. The positive-consultation group consisted of a firm diagnosis. In this group, the patient was told confidently, "This is your diagnosis and you are going to be better in a few days." The negative-consultation group was told the diagnosis was unclear. For example, they might have heard, "We don't know what you have, and we are not sure how long it is going to take before you get better." Interestingly, even though there was no actual treatment difference between the two groups, the positive group experienced significantly faster positive results. This study was actually replicated in a group with acute tonsillitis as well. Based on all these studies, we should confidently and boldly reinforce to our patients a vision of positive progress and eventual results.[65]

A number of examples of enhanced placebo effects have been demonstrated within the musculoskeletal context.

---

64 Barrett, B., Muller, D., Rakel, D., Rabago, D., Marchand, L., and Scheder, J.C. "Placebo, Meaning, and Health." *Perspectives in Biology and Medicine* 49, no. 2 (2006): 178-98. https://doi.org/10.1353/pbm.2006.0019.

65 Olsson, Björn, Olsson, Birgitta, and Tibblin, Gösta. "Effect of Patients Expectations on Recovery from Acute Tonsillitis." *Family Practice* 6, no. 3 (1989): 188-92. https://doi.org/10.1093/fampra/6.3.188.

Koes and colleagues (1992) studied the use of spinal manipulation for cervical and lumbar pain in 256 patients with nonspecific back and neck disorders.[66] They were randomly assigned to four groups and received manual physical therapy, physical therapy, placebo-device therapy (using a "detuned" ultrasonography machine and a "detuned" short-wave diathermy machine with sounds and lights), or treatment from a general practitioner. Six weeks of manual therapy or physical therapy care were both significantly better (by the same margin) than treatment with the sham machines, but the phony machines significantly outperformed care by the general practitioner. It cannot be determined whether the manual and physical therapies had specific treatment effects or stronger placebo effects than the inanimate gadgets. Nonetheless, in this experiment, treatment with sham machines surpassed treatment from a competent physician for relief of low back pain. Perhaps the repeat visits to the physical therapists enhanced patients' relationships with their physical therapists, which, in turn, further engaged interactions and collaborative expectations that positively influenced these outcomes.

The impact of both placebo and nocebo can be startling. One noted researcher conducted a randomized clinical trial involving 270 people who were under treatment

66   Koes, B. W., Bouter, L. M., van Mameren, H., Essers, A. H.M., Verstegen, G. M.J.R., Hofhuizen, D. M., Houben, J. P., and Knipschild, P. G. "The Effectiveness of Manual Therapy, Physiotherapy, and Treatment by the General Practitioner for Nonspecific Back and Neck Complaints." *Spine* 17, no. 1 (1992): 28-35. https://doi.org/10.1097/00007632-199201000-00005.

with severe arm pain—things like carpal tunnel syndrome, chronic shoulder pain, and wrist pain.[67] In one part of the study, half the patients were getting pain-reducing pills and half received acupuncture treatments. Nearly a third of the trial participants were complaining of terrible side effects. Some ultimately reported they felt so sluggish that they couldn't get out of bed. Others said the needles were causing swelling and redness. Another group reported real relief. Interestingly, the pills were made of cornstarch, and the needles were retractable shams that never pierced the skin. The importance of this for us as caregivers is clear: be careful as you can influence what can be perceived as both harmful and positive effects!

Another experiment involved 262 adults with irritable bowel syndrome (IBS).[68] There was a no-treatment control group, a second group that received sham acupuncture without much interaction with the practitioner, and a third group that received sham acupuncture with great attention lavished upon them—at least twenty minutes of what you might consider overly sentimental care. For example, they might hear, "I know how difficult this is for you. This treatment has excellent results." Practitioners were required to

67 Kaptchuk, Ted J., Stason, William B., Davis, Roger B., Legedza, Anna R. T., Schnyer, Rosa N., Kerr, Catherine E., Stone, David A., Nam, Bong Hyun, Kirsch, Irving, and Goldman, Rose H. "Sham Device v Inert Pill: Randomised Controlled Trial of Two Placebo Treatments." *BMJ* 332, no. 7538 (2006): 391-97. https://doi.org/10.1136/bmj.38726.603310.55.

68 Kaptchuk, T.J., Kelley, J.M., Conboy, L.A., Davis, R.B., Kerr, C.E., Jacobson, E.E., Kirsch, I., et al. "Components of Placebo Effect: Randomised Controlled Trial in Patients with Irritable Bowel Syndrome." *BMJ* 336, no. 7651 (2008): 999-1003. https://doi.org/10.1136/bmj.39524.439618.25.

touch the hands or shoulders of members of this third group and spend at least twenty seconds lost in thoughtful silence. The results were not that surprising. The patients who experienced the greatest relief were those who received the most care. Said another way, there was a dose-dependent response even for placebo treatment. Thus, the more care people got, even if it was fake care, the better they tended to do. As detailed previously, the disproportionate time spent on paperwork and regulatory matters robs our patients of more and thus better care. The evidence is compelling; it's time to give back time to healthcare providers who can be more impactful by unleashing such wasteful constraints.

Finally, in a study on aerobic exercise involving participants in a ten-week program, one group was told that the exercise would enhance their aerobic capacity.[69] A second group was told the exercise would enhance their aerobic capacity as well as their psychological well-being. Both groups improved their aerobic capacity but only the second group improved in life satisfaction or psychological well-being. Based on this, when we are communicating with our patients, we need to emphasize the direct benefit to the health condition as well as the additional benefits, such as psychological enhancements.

---

69   Edwards, Steve. "Physical Exercise and Psychological Well-Being." *South African Journal of Psychology* 36, no. 2 (2006): 357-73. https://doi.org/10.1177/008124630603600209.

Beware of the Nocebo Impact

Language can also create *negative* effects, as noted in a recent study by Lin and colleagues (2013). The authors reported on an Aboriginal Australian population previously at low risk of chronic low back pain. They discovered that advice from healthcare providers, emphasizing strictly biological or anatomical issues, like posture or their spinal structure solely from radiographic imaging, resulted in the patients having negative beliefs, a pessimistic outlook, and greater disability.[70]

A nocebo response also influences provider interactions and usually in unintended ways. In an experimental study designed in part to measure fear-avoidance behavior, fifty patients with chronic back pain were randomly divided into two groups prior to the performance of leg flexion tests.[71] One group was informed that the test could lead to a slight increase in pain, while the other group was told that the test was painless. The former group reported stronger pain and performed fewer leg flexion repetitions than the group that received neutral instruction. Words do indeed mean things, and, as Called to Care providers, we have to

70 Lin, Ivan B., Osullivan, Peter B., Coffin, Juli A., Mak, Donna B., Toussaint, Sandy, and Straker, Leon M. "Disabling Chronic Low Back Pain as an Iatrogenic Disorder: A Qualitative Study in Aboriginal Australians." *BMJ Open* 3, no. 4 (2013): e002654–e002654. https://doi.org/10.1136/bmjopen-2013-002654.

71 Pfingsten, Michael, Leibing, Eric, Harter, Wulf, Kröner-Herwig, Birgit, Hempel, Doreen, Kronshage, Uta, and Hildebrandt, Jan. "Fear-Avoidance Behavior and Anticipation of Pain in Patients with Chronic Low Back Pain: A Randomized Controlled Study." *Pain Medicine* 2, no. 4 (2001): 259–66. https://doi.org/10.1046/j.1526-4637.2001.01044.x.

control what we may view as innocuous—for example, the phrase "a slight increase in pain" as what we say can have far-reaching implications.

How We Can Use Meaning to Magnify the Power of Placebo

This all demonstrates that a placebo response is not all in one's head, so to speak; instead, it is a phenomenon that catalyzes neurobiological responses that influence objectively measurable outcomes. Key placebo phenomena that contribute to quantifiable outcomes are conveyed via practitioner behaviors during clinical care. They may be optimized when a clinician's wish to do good meets the patient's desire to be helped;[72] here the art and science of medicine work together via a mixture of practitioner framing and evidence-based interventions.

Moerman and Jonas (2002) have suggested thinking about placebo in a new and different way—one that could help clinicians promote desired positive effects. They explain their contention by analyzing two studies. In the first, a group of medical students was asked to participate in a study on two new drugs: a tranquilizer and a stimulant. Each student was given a packet containing either one or two blue or

72   Sanderson, Christine, Hardy, Janet, Spruyt, Odette, and Currow, David C. "Placebo and Nocebo Effects in Randomized Controlled Trials: The Implications for Research and Practice." *Journal of Pain and Symptom Management* 46, no. 5 (2013): 722–30. https://doi.org/10.1016/j.jpainsymman.2012.12.005.

red tablets.[73] They were not told that the tablets were inert and contained no medicine. After taking the tablets, their questionnaire responses indicated that the red tablets acted as stimulants while the blue ones acted as depressants and that two tablets had a greater effect than one. The students were not responding to the inert tablets. Instead, they were responding to "meanings" in the experiment, specifically that red generally means up, hot, or danger, while blue means down, cool, or quiet, and that two pills would be twice as strong as one.

Also, in a randomized controlled trial,[74] female patients with headaches received one of four medications: aspirin in a package displaying a widely advertised brand name, aspirin in a plain package, a placebo marked with the same widely advertised brand name, or an unmarked placebo. In this study, branded aspirin worked better than unbranded aspirin, which worked better than branded placebo, which worked better than the unbranded placebo.

The authors clarify that the "placebo effect" is a result of physiological changes in the patient caused by assigning meaning to the treatment—the association of the color

73 Moerman, D. E., and Jonas, W. B. "Deconstructing the Placebo Effect and Finding the Meaning Response." *Annals of Internal Medicine* 136, no. 6 (2002): 471-76. https://doi.org/doi:10.7326/0003-4819-136-6-200203190-00011.

74 Branthwaite, A., and Cooper, P. "Analgesic Effects of Branding in Treatment of Headaches." *BMJ (Clinical Research Edition)* 282, no. 6276 (1981): 1576-78. https://doi.org/10.1136/bmj.282.6276.1576.

red with stimulation, of blue with coolness, and of well-known brands with efficacy. They suggest calling this effect a *meaning* response. Meaning responses elicited after the use of inert or sham treatments can be called "placebo effect" when desirable and "nocebo effect" when not.

So, what does this mean for all of us?

We've learned previously that clinician mannerisms (enthusiastic or lukewarm), language (positive or negative), as well as appropriate persuasion techniques (framing and refocusing) impart meaning to patients and can influence outcomes.[75] By "meaning" we are specifically referring to interpretation and all of the perceived consequences of that meaning. For example, if a physician says to you, "I'm going to clean up your messy joint through knee arthroscopy," would that have a different impact than saying, "We're going to prescribe an anti-inflammatory that will inhibit the production of prostaglandins, which are involved in inflammatory processes"? Interestingly, surgery has a significant meaning response that can vary greatly based on one's experiences, and, not surprisingly, a significant component of surgery is, in fact, the placebo effect. But it is the *clarity* of the language (e.g., "cleaning up a messy knee") that really makes sense to patients, and this is what

75 Swindell, J. S., Mcguire, A. L., and Halpern, S. D. "Beneficent Persuasion: Techniques and Ethical Guidelines to Improve Patients Decisions." *The Annals of Family Medicine* 8, no. 3 (2010): 260-64. https://doi.org/10.1370/afm.1118.

we have to keep in mind. It is easy to default into medical jargon but the Called to Care practitioner, by maintaining a patient perspective approach, communicates with clarity.

By embracing the science of placebo, healthcare professionals are ideally suited to positively influence the meaning response through communication, treatment expectations, and even considering clinic design, attire, and atmosphere, all of which also have been shown to have an effect.

Actionable Steps

The following methods can serve as a checklist that will enhance the placebo while limiting nocebo.

Leverage a collaborative model of shared decision-making: This enables a patient to have a sense of control and ownership of therapeutic decisions and the overall process. This enhanced autonomy increases perceived ownership of the shared plan, nurtures the therapeutic alliance, and makes adherence and engagement with the treatment more likely.[76] The therapeutic alliance and treatment plan should take into account both specific and nonspecific treatment effects, meaning the understanding that all of the treatment interventions have a stated goal but being mindful of other consequences from the direct goal,

---

76   Data-Franco, João, and Berk, Michael. "The Nocebo Effect: A Clinicians Guide." *Australian & New Zealand Journal of Psychiatry* 47, no. 7 (2012): 617-23. https://doi.org/10.1177/0004867412464717.

some of which can be positive and others negative. This combination effect, when married with careful monitoring of outcomes over time, will ensure improvement and avoid potential unintended consequences.[77]

Positive framing: Imagine that you are about to get a flu vaccine and the nurse says, "The majority of people tolerate this well, they go right back to work, and they have no ill effects from this vaccine." Alternatively, imagine the nurse saying, "This might cause a headache, you might have to miss a day of work, and you might get a fever." The results overwhelmingly demonstrate that the second group develops these adverse effects. Always consider this when relaying key data to patients. For example, you might say, "The great majority of patients who have what you have tolerate this treatment and do great." When you say the opposite (e.g., that "5 percent of our patients report severe side effects"), patients focus on that 5 percent and consider themselves part of that group.

Shape expectations: The most important question you can ask your patient is, "What is your expectation?" Supportive research has demonstrated that shaping expectations is a precursor to a positive outcome. Understanding expectations from the perspective of the patient is insightful as the

---

77   Bootzin, Richard R., and Bailey, Elaine T. "Understanding Placebo, Nocebo, and Iatrogenic Treatment Effects." *Journal of Clinical Psychology* 61, no. 7 (2005): 871–80. https://doi.org/10.1002/jclp.20131.

ranges of experiences are broad and often counterintuitive to the provider. Questioning and clarifying, as well as setting agreements, leaves a patient with clarity, confidence, and understanding.

Patient preferences: Interestingly enough, patient preference has been shown, in some research cycles, as being equivalent to placebo in regard to positive patient outcome influence. If a patient comes to you with such a strong preference for a certain technique, unless it is harmful, you would be hard-pressed not to do it. The research supports preferences in exercise and diet programs, and it influences outcomes. Providing strong evidence-based interventions alongside patient preferences particularly in the early course of treatment is very comforting in patient-centered care. Remember, placebo or techniques that influence have a physical implication. It is important to not reflexively default to all this "being in a patient's head."

Encourage adherence: Simply taking medicine sends a signal to the body that we are doing something good, and it has a strong and powerful physiologic effect demonstrated in numerous studies. Consider the fact that when researchers measure adherence in terms of medication, it is usually whether or not a pill is taken 80 percent of the time, so remind patients that adherence is critical but that missing a few doses will not negate its effect. This reinforcement is a further example of influencing a placebo effect. Furthermore, in cardiac research, studies are often conducted over many years. In one study on beta-blockers, five-year (or more) adherers had a mortality rate that was equivalent to a placebo group of five-year adherers.

Avoid using negative words: Certain words have to be eliminated in our patient conversations. A study on patients receiving injections of radiographic substances indicated that anxiety and pain were heightened by the use of negative words like sting, burn, hurt, bad, and pain when explaining the procedure or expressing sympathy. In another study, the person injecting a local anesthetic before the induction of epidural anesthesia in women about to give birth said, "We're going to give you a local anesthetic that will numb the area so you will be comfortable during the procedure." Alternatively, patients were told, "You're going feel a big bee sting; this is the worst part of the procedure." The perceived pain was significantly greater with the latter statement.

Other Factors that Impact the Placebo Effect

It's interesting to note that in Brazil, the placebo effect is about 7 percent; in Germany, the effect is 59 percent, which is about twice as high as in the rest of the world. Also, a gene has been identified that tells the practitioner or researcher whether there is a susceptibility to placebo with certain afflictions such as depression. Think about how beneficial this is to drug companies performing clinical research.

Furthermore, there is no real difference between men and women relative to their propensity to be influenced by placebo; however, they are influenced differently. For women, it is through conditioning. In studies of chemotherapy, if women take a lemon-juice drink with the chemo, they begin to associate the two and have nausea and vomiting with just the sight and smell of the lemon juice. This can be used in a positive way; for example, if you have had a positive effect from a visit to a physical therapist, you are more likely to associate that in a conditioning way for future visits.

Men are most susceptible to the shaping of expectations. Men like to be told what to do and what to expect. For example, consider a large study on benign prostatic hyperplasia (BPH). Men who were given drugs were put into two groups. One group was told that they would have various sexual dysfunctions; a second group was not told anything. As you can imagine, the group that was told they would have dysfunction had it three-to-one over the group that did not.

So, we need to embrace the placebo and nonspecific effects via shaping expectations, being positive, framing in a positive way, monitoring and adherence, and understanding how to negate the nocebo. Healthcare practitioners worldwide would benefit from further study on the methods that enhance meaning effects (e.g., positivity, problem framing, patient engagement, and the use of ritual) and utilize them as therapeutic adjuncts in which the patients' preferences are maximized for positive outcomes.

Of course, many of us are likely already employing some of these strategies without realizing there is sound science behind them. However, the evolving science suggests that it is time to broaden our knowledge to better leverage and employ such techniques with the goal of promoting more positive outcomes in our patients through influencing placebo while also negating a nocebo effect.

For more resources on this topic, visit CalledtoCarebook. com.

CHAPTER SEVEN

PEAK-END RULE

THE SCIENCE BEHIND "ENDING ON A HIGH NOTE"

"All's well that ends well."

—SHAKESPEARE

Imagine getting a call close to the holidays from your child's school. He has injured himself during football practice. Although you are up against a work deadline, you have to find an available doctor, leave work early, pick up your son, battle traffic under gloomy skies, hunt for a parking space at the physician's office, and sign in by 5:30 p.m. to ensure your son gets to see the doctor that evening. Fortunately, you are pleased to discover the doctor is personable, running on time, and able to see your son immediately. Amy, who is introduced to you as your personal concierge, checks you in efficiently.

The visit goes well, and you are satisfied with the doctor's level of care. However, you are then met with a higher-than-expected bill and are confused about the limitations of your co-pay. You anticipate a chilling response and experience to your genuine concerns. You make the call to the office, and Amy is attentive and amiable. She somewhat surprises you by first asking and showing genuine concern for your son. She even wants to know about the football season. She is responsive and listens carefully. She offers to research the issue and promises that during your follow-up visit, there will be less time spent on insurance hassles. She ends the call expressing her personal commitment to take full responsibility for all the issues brought up and offers an additional promise to reach back to you within three days.

Two days later, you get a follow-up call that addresses your questions and includes a direct phone number for any future concerns about any aspect of care you may need in the future. You quickly shift from feeling frustration to experiencing gratitude. You understand what you are responsible for paying, and you immediately schedule a follow-up visit for your son. Your anticipated experience is now overwhelmed by a positive actual experience that will be remembered well into the future.

What You Need to Know about the Peak-End Rule

Daniel Kahneman and his colleagues have shown that how

we remember our past experiences is almost entirely determined by two things:

1. The average of how the experience felt when at its peak (best or worst)
2. How the experience felt when it ended

This is known as the peak-end rule, and it is what we use to summarize our experiences. We rely on the summary to later remind ourselves of how the experience felt. This, in turn, affects our decisions about whether to have that experience again.

Interestingly, related research demonstrates that the duration of an experienced episode has minimal influence on the affective memory of it. This is known as "duration neglect."[78] Research has been replicated in clinical situations and has confirmed that people tend to remember the rising and falling trends of their pain and that pain levels at the end of treatment are recalled more readily than average or peak pain.[79] In other research in clinical settings, patients' memories of pain during uncomfortable procedures were a function of their peak experiences and the

78 Kahneman, Daniel, Fredrickson, Barbara L., Schreiber, Charles A., and Redelmeier, Donald A. "When More Pain Is Preferred to Less: Adding a Better End." *Psychological Science* 4, no. 6 (1993): 401–5. https://doi.org/10.1111/j.1467-9280.1993.tb00589.x.

79 Ariely, Dan, and Carmon, Ziv. "Gestalt Characteristics of Experiences: The Defining Features of Summarized Events." *Journal of Behavioral Decision Making* 13, no. 2 (2000): 191–201. https://doi.org/10.1002/(sici)1099-0771(200004/06)13:2<191::aid-bdm330>3.0.co;2-a.

pain experienced in the last three minutes of a procedure. Furthermore, the length of the procedure was not particularly impactful on experience.[80]

These findings can enable us to improve the patient's experience. In the case of our theoretical story about your son's football accident and subsequent doctor visit, the experience ended with a positive follow-up call. But we can also impact the visit itself. During an interesting lab study, participants were asked to listen to a pair of very loud and unpleasant noises via headphones. One noise lasted for eight seconds; the other lasted for sixteen seconds. The first eight seconds of the second noise were identical to the first noise, whereas the second eight seconds, while still loud and unpleasant, were not as loud as the first eight seconds. Later, the participants were told they would have to listen to one of the noises again and they could choose which one. Clearly, the second noise was worse—it lasted twice as long. Nonetheless, the overwhelming majority chose the second to be repeated.

Why? Whereas both noises were unpleasant and had the same aversive peak, the second had a less unpleasant ending so it was remembered as less annoying than the first. Likewise, if you are having a tooth drilled, you will

---

80 Redelmeier, Donald A., and Kahneman, Daniel. "Patients' Memories of Painful Medical Treatments: Real-Time and Retrospective Evaluations of Two Minimally Invasive Procedures." *Pain* 66, no. 1 (1996): 3–8. https://doi.org/10.1016/0304-3959(96)02994-6.

find it less painful if the dentist ends the procedure with some lightening of the drill's intensity. And, interestingly, we don't only approach our experiences of pleasure and pain this way; one study found that participants who were given free DVDs said they were more pleased with the gifts if they received the popular ones after the less popular ones than if they had received the exact same DVDs in the opposite order.

In another study, participants were asked to hold their hands in painfully cold water until they were invited to remove them and offered warm towels. During the immersion, they were asked to provide a continuous record of the pain they experienced. Each participant experienced two cold-hand episodes; some started with a short episode and some started with a long one. The short episode consisted of immersion for sixty seconds at 57°F followed by a warm cloth and a seven-minute break. The long episode, conducted, on the other hand, consisted of the short episode plus thirty additional seconds; however, the water was made 34°F warmer and without the knowledge of the participant. The difference was barely perceptible.

After completing both episodes, participants were told that they needed to perform a third trial and were given the choice to repeat either the first or second experience. They had no explicit knowledge that the duration of each episode was different or that the water temperature had changed.

The peak-end rule predicted a worse memory of the short episode; duration neglect predicted that the difference between sixty and ninety seconds would be ignored. This is exactly what the researchers found. Eighty percent of participants chose to repeat the long episode and endure thirty seconds of slightly reduced but totally needless pain.[81]

In perhaps the most relevant and quite remarkable example of the peak-end rule in operation, men undergoing diagnostic colonoscopy exams were asked to report on how they felt moment by moment during the exam and how they felt when it was over. Two decades ago, most people found these exams to be quite unpleasant—so much so that many avoided getting regular tests altogether. During this particular test, both groups of patients had standard colonoscopies; however, the doctor left the instrument in place within the second group of patients for a short time. This was still unpleasant but much less so because the scope was not moving. Thus, the second group experienced the same moment-by-moment discomfort as the first group of patients with the addition of somewhat lesser discomfort for an additional twenty seconds at the end. Shortly after the experiment was over, the second group rated their experience as less unpleasant than did the first. Whereas both

81   Finn, Bridgid. "Ending on a High Note: Adding a Better End to Effortful Study." *Journal of Experimental Psychology: Learning, Memory, and Cognition* 36, no. 6 (2010): 1548–53. https://doi.org/10.1037/a0020605.

groups had the same peak experience, the second group had a milder experience at the end.[82]

This made a difference. Over a five-year period after the exam, patients in the second group were more likely to comply with the call for a follow-up colonoscopy. Since they recalled their experiences as being less unpleasant, they were less inclined to avoid them in the future. Therefore, the total amount of pain was well predicted by the average level of pain reported at the worst moment of the experience and at the end. The duration of the procedure had no effect whatsoever on the rating of overall pain.[83]

How We Can Use the Peak-End Rule to Create Positivity

The peak-end rule has enormous significance for those of us in the healthcare industry since so many aspects of a patient's care can induce temporary pain and discomfort. Let's also remember that all of the positive psychology techniques and interventions work together to impact outcome clinically and away from the healthcare environment. Peak-end cannot replace high-quality connection, appropriate use of positivity, empathy, self-efficacy, and active con-

82 Fredrickson, Barbara L., and Kahneman, Daniel. "Duration Neglect in Retrospective Evaluations of Affective Episodes." *Journal of Personality and Social Psychology* 65, no. 1 (1993): 45–55. https://doi.org/10.1037/0022-3514.65.1.45.

83 Redelmeier, D.A., Katz, J., and Kahneman, D. "Memories of Colonoscopy: A Randomized Trial." *Pain* 104, no. 1-2 (2003): 187–94. https://doi.org/10.1016/s0304-3959(03)00003-4.

structure communication. For this reason, we need to be frequently reminded that all of these are clinical skills that have to be refined through appropriate mentoring, deliberative feedback, and accountability.

At the most basic level, we can prioritize high-quality interactions, excellent customer service skills, and other tactics to enhance patients' visits. Such tactics might include:

- The creation of a high-energy, positive, and upbeat atmosphere
- An extreme emphasis on friendliness and levity
- Efficient administrative services
- A culture of commitment to exceeding patient expectations and giving priority to patient needs

The peak-end rule's applicability is truly amazing. We could apply this knowledge by working to ensure more treatments and tests end in pleasant or less painful ways. For example, physical therapists know that hands-on care via manual therapies and passive stretching exercises are key evidence-based procedures that restore range of motion, joint integrity, and produce longer-term pain reduction and functional recovery.[84] However, these procedures can be very painful. The research suggests that the procedures should be elongated with the majority of discomfort at the

---

84 Di Fabio, Richard P. "Efficacy of Manual Therapy." *Physical Therapy* 72, no. 12 (1992): 853–64. https://doi.org/10.1093/ptj/72.12.853.

beginning, and there should progressively be less discomfort and eventually comfort. This may be achieved with gentle oscillations; also, patients could be kept apprised of positive gains associated with the procedure. Additionally, each physical therapy visit could end with a "What went well?" discussion, which ensures peaks are revisited.

We could also accomplish this by celebrating milestone events and discharges. For example, let's say you often treat patients over longer intervals of time (as we often do in physical therapy). At the end of the process, you could issue T-shirts or fun diplomas. You might further influence positive memories by sending handwritten thank-you notes to patients after discharge. This strengthens relationships and impacts patients' overall memories of working with your healthcare practice.

As Called to Care healthcare practitioners, let's make it a priority to end all interactions with our patients on a high note—that is, what is remembered, recalled, and savored.

For more resources on this topic, visit CalledtoCarebook. com.

CHAPTER EIGHT

PUTTING THE *PATIENT* BACK INTO PATIENT CARE

"What patients seek is not scientific knowledge that doctors hide but existential authenticity each person must find on her own. Getting too deeply into statistics is like trying to quench a thirst with salty water. The angst of facing mortality has no remedy in probability."

—PAUL KALANITHI

Five patients in a row with flu-like symptoms—fast onset of fever and chills, muscle aches, and some accompanying runny nose and watery eyes. Dr. Blain had gotten so used to the diagnosis that he had gone from a fifteen-minute patient interaction on the first patient of the day to less than three minutes on the third. An overrun waiting room and an already overworked staff made it impossible for Dr. Blain to take a break or to even differentiate between patients—they all were the same. By patient three, the story was so similar that Dr. Blain stopped listening; by the fifth patient, he even became bored. At that point, he stopped, removed himself from the office, and went for a few-minute walk, took a few mindful breaths, and then returned. Dr. Blain understood that the natural process of calcification or dehumanization was occurring, and this was not good for him or his patients.

Remembering the Patient's Experience

Imagine how many times an internist will diagnose patients with flu viruses, colds, bronchitis, strep throat, and other health concerns in the depth of winter. Still, every time a new patient comes in the door, it is so important to treat him or her like an individual with unique concerns. This means taking the time to listen to patients, being present in the moment, and showing concern for their individual needs. Of course, this can be difficult to sustain consistently amid the demands of modern-day medicine. In fact, one of the key challenges in healthcare today is remembering the *patient* in patient care.

This all begins with the reminder and the need to constantly revisit that there are two fundamental components to the initial encounter:

1. Each patient is genuinely, authentically, and remarkably unique with individual perspectives, experiences, and thoughts.
2. Your examination routine or ritual, while not new to you, is very much a new experience for the patient.

Often, we forget the new and unique nature of these two components and begin to compartmentalize every patient into a diagnosis pattern, and thus we commoditize the new encounter rather than use it as an opportunity to cement caring, compassion, and empathy from the initial greeting of the patient. Remembering you're treating Mr. Smith and not Mr. Smith's knees and considering patients' emotional needs when conducting routine exams and tests, entering exam rooms, presenting routine diagnoses, and responding to routine questions is a reinvigoration habit that energizes the Called to Care practitioner.

As the professions within healthcare have evolved, the stakeholders have expanded greatly. A significant part of the healthcare challenge is that the payor, oftentimes the government in terms of Medicare and Medicaid, and private payors like United Healthcare and Aetna have inserted processes and outsourced agencies between themselves and the provider. In effect, this has created superimposed processes and regulatory requirements that literally detract from time spent with patients. Providers have, in real terms, seen their payments reduced and their paperwork requirements go up, which adds cost to the process thus further reducing reimbursements for services. To oversimplify, industry-wide fears, uncertainties, and changes drive today's healthcare professionals to replace care, compassion, and empathy with compliance and adherence to these demands, including prescriptive care, which is referred to as "cookbook medicine." This tough environment is difficult to overcome with the most daunting challenge being that every patient interaction must be treated with the utmost care and concern regardless of the background; information and diagnoses must be carefully conveyed in a manner that supports the notion that this is the first time the patient has heard your expertise.

The Concepts of Calcification, Dehumanization, and Decalcification

A technique we use in *Called to Care* is called regular *decalcification*, which is based on a concept utilized in the customer service industry, particularly those who work in call centers. As you can imagine, call-center employees are often in contact with unhappy customers and a lot of negativity. After all, few of us think of calling our phone, internet, or cable company intermittently to tell them how good our service was on a certain day. This disproportionate exposure to the bad means that *calcification* or becoming numb to human connections and emotions ensues and *dehumanization* can set in. Employees can become hardened toward customers and treat them as two-dimensional objects rather than three-dimensional humans. This frequently results in contentious, unhappy dynamics between businesses and customers. Decalcification involves any type of routine, habit, or ritual that enables us to stop and remind ourselves that we are dealing with fellow human beings and restores connection and thus humanity.

Dehumanization in healthcare is quite similar. It's simply impossible to deliver exceptional experiences or care when you have dehumanized your customer or patient. In most cases, the culprit is the simple process of good people temporarily turning patients and customers into two-dimensional objects. Forgetting, just for a moment, that the primary focus is the patient (a human being with expressed and unexpressed needs) and not simply the diagnosis (osteoarthritis of the knee).

We know that *how* and *when* we begin to calcify (or dehumanize) turns out to be highly variable and dependent upon both individual and institutional factors. In some cases, when we are bombarded by tough patients, rules, healthcare obstacles, and complaints, healthcare employees need to decalcify as often as every four hours—especially healthcare providers. Additionally, there is some research showing that physicians start to dehumanize, in general, by the time they have left medical school.[85] Of note, dehuman-

85 Newton, Bruce W., Barber, Laurie, Clardy, James, Cleveland, Elton, and O'Sullivan, Patricia. "Is There Hardening of the Heart during Medical School?" *Academic Medicine* 83, no. 3 (2008): 244–49. https://doi.org/10.1097/acm.0b013e3181637837.

ization or calcification occurs naturally and transitionally, unlike burnout, which manifests as a complex affect that includes loss of zest, purpose, and meaning in your work.

To better understand the process of calcification, we need an understanding of construal level theory (CLT). According to CLT, the further psychologically I am from a problem or an object, the more abstract I think about it; thus, the more likely it is for calcification to set in. Conversely, the closer I am psychologically to a problem or an object, the more concretely I think about it and the less likely it is for calcification to set in.

As an example, let's say I ask you about a vacation you are planning to take in five years. I say, "Describe for me what the vacation will look like." You might talk about how the destination is relaxing, sunny, has many beaches, and is far away; these are all obviously very big-picture concepts. However, if I said to you the day before you are leaving on a vacation, "What are you thinking?" you might say, "Well, did I print my boarding pass? What time do I need to get to the airport? I can't wait to get to the hotel." These are obviously all very concrete details.

If you are a physical therapy student and I ask you about how you are going to prepare for your future patients, you might say, "I'm going to study hard, do good clinical rotations, and apply the evidence that I learn." Now let's say you *are* a licensed physical therapist and I ask how you are going to prepare for your patients. You might say, "Well, I would look at my schedule, make sure that I have my equipment, and stay current on the rules and regulations." Again, these are very concrete details. In essence, the process of calcification occurs when we begin to psychologically see or remove the patient from the process of care and instead ascribe diagnoses separate and away from the act of treatment or caring.

How You Can Manage Calcification

You can mitigate the potential for calcification in many ways. You might review your patients' goals before you examine them. You might also sit down with them every visit and talk with them about some things *other* than their health concerns to remind yourself that they are unique human beings like yourself. The key to managing the calcification process is to simply avoid focusing too much on the objective details, facts, and figures that force you into dehumanizing your patient. Said differently, when we fall into the trap of "objectifying" the patient—How old are you? When did you get hurt? How did you get hurt? Have you ever been hurt before?—rather than mixing subjective and unrelated conversations into the encounter, we move toward calcifying and dehumanizing.

We refer to the term resiliency as the ability to overcome

challenges and bounce back stronger, wiser, and more learned. Resiliency has been studied extensively and broadly tells us that being aware of and understanding the triggers that influence a behavior along with training in cognitive behavioral therapy are critical to accomplishing resiliency. In the context of patient care, sensing when dehumanizing is occurring—like making every patient's diagnosis routine, only asking objective questions, becoming somewhat bored—are triggers for us that calcification is taking its toll. Like Dr. Blain in our opening story, when we feel a trigger, this should prompt us to ask subjective questions, take a time-out, take some deep breaths, or use whatever coping mechanisms that work and that ultimately move us to mitigate (and ideally reverse) this process.

Some suggested personal routines that manage calcification and promote relaxation or that "hack the brain" and reverse the process include:

- Taking frequent breaks, including walking or something physical that changes the posture and actions from caregiver
- Listening to music that enables distraction from the clinic environment
- Enjoying the aroma of flowers or something that taps into the sense of smell
- Looking at pictures, particularly those that evoke memories

- Meditation or other exercises in mindfulness. Research on meditation is shedding light on its many benefits, including the ability to accept the feelings associated with calcification, not try to fight them, and instead let them pass through nonjudgmental focus and purposeful attention.

In our experience, it is highly personal as to the frequency and length of these breaks. Some practitioners can go on for hours without calcification while others begin at forty minutes. The key insight is to "know thyself" and use whatever mechanisms that work for you. Calcification and burnout have a very fast antidote, but it takes the experience, sensitivity, and the vulnerability to acknowledge this very real phenomenon and the intention to put into place practices that eliminate it.

How We Can Put the Patient Back in Our Picture

Healthcare providers and caregivers are blessed to work in an environment of meaningful, purposeful work. However, distractions and externalities do harden us of the joy and fulfilling work that we do. This phenomenon is normal, but thankfully, we have a host of antidotes at our hand, including awareness. Managing the symptoms that occur in us is paramount to managing our patients as our behavior directly influences their care and experience. A side-by-side strategy to managing dehumanization is to be reminded frequently of why you became a healthcare practitioner. It is helpful to save and regularly review the thank-you notes, pictures, and testimonials sent by patients, which remind us of how we impact patients in meaningful ways and return them to activities, sports, work, and recovery.

For more resources on this topic, visit CalledtoCarebook. com.

CHAPTER NINE

GRATITUDE

THE SCIENCE BEHIND THANKFULNESS

"Gratitude is the healthiest of all human emotions. The more you express gratitude for what you have, the more likely you will have even more to express gratitude for."

—ZIG ZIGLAR

In many parts of the country, February can be a particularly dreary time of year. Landscapes are often brown under overcast skies, the days are short, and flu season takes hold. Therefore, this can be a particularly challenging time of year for those of us in healthcare, especially as we deal with weather delays, school breaks, and health challenges in our own families and lives. However, we must continue to treat our patients with the utmost care and concern, and a key tool for doing so dovetails with the reason for the season: *gratitude*. While many of the key interventions presented in this book are those used directly on patients, gratitude, like sensing dehumanization, is included for a Called to Care provider because it impacts our mindset and enables us to be better providers. We can't improve our ability to take care of patients unless we use evidence-based resources that optimize us, and gratitude is one of them.

The History and Science of Gratitude

Throughout history, many cultures have regarded the experience and expression of gratitude as beneficial for individuals and society, as evidenced by its inclusion as a character strength that has been valued across religions and philosophies for centuries.[86] In addition, trait gratitude is one of the top three strengths that predict happiness and life satisfaction, or what is often referred to as subjective well-being.[87] Research on gratitude also suggests it is a key element for sparking positive change.[88] Furthermore, gratitude has been found to reduce feelings of envy, make our memories happier, and help us experience more good

---

86 Peterson, Christopher, and Seligman, Martin E. P. *Character Strengths and Virtues: A Handbook and Classification*. Washington, DC: American Psychological Association/Oxford University Press, 2004.

87 Park, N., Peterson, C., and Seligman, M.E.P. "Strengths of Character and Well-Being." *Journal of Social and Clinical Psychology* 23, no. 5 (2004): 603-19. https://doi.org/10.1521/jscp.23.5.603.50748.

88 Bono, G., Emmons, R., and McCullough, M.E. "Gratitude in Practice and the Practice of Gratitude." In *Positive Psychology in Practice*, edited by P.A. Linley and S. Joseph, 464-81. Hoboken, NJ: Wiley, 2004.

feelings and bounce back from stress. The emotions of appreciation and gratitude are shown to introduce a relaxation response, slow depressive symptoms, and correlate significantly with vitality and energy.

Consider, for example, the emotional and physical well-being of those who have won the lottery versus those who keep a gratitude journal. Over a period of time, those who keep a gratitude journal come out on top. Some particularly interesting research on gratitude has focused on its impact on family caregivers (spouses) of Alzheimer's patients. Alzheimer's is a particularly pernicious disease since it can ravage both mind and body, progress at very different rates, vary in terms of its symptoms, follow an up-and-down trajectory, and progressively require around-the-clock care. This can have an enormous impact on a caregiver's physical and mental well-being. Toward the end of this disease, family members find themselves adapting to the constant changes of care required and often need the assistance of strangers via a nursing home. In one experiment, a group of caregivers utilized gratitude journals on a daily basis while another group did not; those utilizing the journal benefited in a myriad of ways (e.g., less stress and less depression).[89]

---

89 Emmons, Robert A. *Thanks! How Practicing Gratitude Can Make You Happier*. New York: Mariner Books / Houghton Mifflin Co., 2008.

How Gratitude Can Help You to Help Others

Gratitude was incorporated into *Called to Care* primarily to assist practitioners in maintaining their own well-being and for its contribution to many facets of patient care (e.g., positivity and empathy). Gratitude can come in many forms. An example seldom seen in the healthcare field, where patients are not viewed as customers, is the gratitude that you express toward a patient for merely showing up and choosing you! They have other options. Patients can sense your thankfulness and a mutual regard is quickly obtained. When medical practitioners are grateful, this resonance transcends to patients and coworkers. A comforting environment and outcomes for patients are facilitated simply by an attitude of gratitude.

Healthcare is all about helping others, and researchers have conceptualized gratitude as an emotion that is always directed toward appreciating the helpful actions of others.[90] Additionally, we know that grateful people experience more positive emotions, have greater life satisfaction, and are more hopeful about the future compared to ungrateful people.[91] Furthermore, highly grateful people

---

90 Mccullough, Michael E., Kilpatrick, Shelley D., Emmons, Robert A., and Larson, David B. "Is Gratitude a Moral Affect?" *Psychological Bulletin* 127, no. 2 (2001): 249–66. https://doi.org/10.1037/0033-2909.127.2.249.

91 Emmons, Robert A., and Mccullough, Michael E. "Counting Blessings versus Burdens: An Experimental Investigation of Gratitude and Subjective Well-Being in Daily Life." *Journal of Personality and Social Psychology* 84, no. 2 (2003): 377–89. https://doi.org/10.1037/0022-3514.84.2.377.

are more empathetic, forgiving, and supportive, as well as less likely to be depressed, anxious, and jealous.[92]

Not only is gratitude strongly associated with happiness, but experimental manipulations of gratitude have been shown to enhance well-being[93] as well as creativity[94] and problem solving[95]—all of these are keys to better clinical decision-making.[96] There have, in fact, been many studies exploring the link between gratitude and well-being. For example, participants in one study were asked to write down five things for which they are grateful once a week for ten weeks; another group was asked to list five daily hassles.[97] The results were impressive: relative to the control group, the participants who expressed gratitude felt

92   Mccullough, Michael E., Tsang, Jo-Ann, and Emmons, Robert A. "Gratitude in Intermediate
     Affective Terrain: Links of Grateful Moods to Individual Differences and Daily Emotional
     Experience." *Journal of Personality and Social Psychology* 86, no. 2 (2004): 295-309. https://doi.
     org/10.1037/0022-3514.86.2.295.

93   Watkins, P.C., Van Gelder, M., and Frias, A. "Furthering the Science of Gratitude." In *Oxford
     Handbook of Positive Psychology*, edited by C.R. Snyder and S.J. Lopez, 2nd ed., 437-45. New York:
     Oxford University Press, 2009.

94   Froh, Jeffrey J., Sefick, William J., and Emmons, Robert A. "Counting Blessings in Early
     Adolescents: An Experimental Study of Gratitude and Subjective Well-Being." *Journal of School
     Psychology* 46, no. 2 (2008): 213-33. https://doi.org/10.1016/j.jsp.2007.03.005.

95   Emmons, R.A. "Gratitude, Subjective Well-Being, and the Brain." In *The Science of Subjective Well-
     Being*, edited by M. Eid and R.J. Larsen, 469-89. New York: Guilford Press, 2008.

96   Estrada, Carlos A., Isen, Alice M., and Young, Mark J. "Positive Affect Improves Creative Problem
     Solving and Influences Reported Source of Practice Satisfaction in Physicians." *Motivation and
     Emotion* 18, no. 4 (1994): 285-99. https://doi.org/10.1007/bf02856470.

97   Emmons, Robert A., and Mccullough. Michael E. "Counting Blessings versus Burdens:
     An Experimental Investigation of Gratitude and Subjective Well-Being in Daily
     Life." *Journal of Personality and Social Psychology* 84, no. 2 (2003): 377-89. https://doi.
     org/10.1037/0022-3514.84.2.377.

more optimistic and more satisfied with their lives. Even their health received a boost; they reported fewer physical symptoms (e.g., headache, acne, coughing, and nausea) and more time spent exercising. A study on internet-based interventions showed that participants who were randomized into the "three good things in life" exercise (they were asked to write down three things that went well—and the reasons why—every night for a week) reported increased happiness and decreased depressive symptoms for six months.[98]

Seligman, Rashid, and Parks (2006) showed the benefits of the blessings exercise in depressed patients. Human beings are naturally biased toward focusing on (and remembering) the negative, which is further exacerbated by depression. The aim of the blessings exercise is to refocus the patient's attention, memory, and expectations away from the negative and toward the positive. They theorize that the blessings exercise is effective because it counteracts a tendency toward excessively focusing on negative events, which contributes to depression.[99] Furthermore, Lyubomirsky (2007) describes the numerous ways that gratitude boosts happiness: it promotes the savoring of life experiences, bolsters self-worth, helps people cope with stress

98 Seligman, Martin E. P., Steen, Tracy A., Park, Nansook, and Peterson, Christopher. "Positive Psychology Progress: Empirical Validation of Interventions." *American Psychologist* 60, no. 5 (2005): 410–21. https://doi.org/10.1037/0003-066x.60.5.410.

99 Seligman, M.E.P., Rashid, T., and Parks, A.C. "Positive Psychotherapy." *American Psychologist* 61, no. 8 (2006): 774–88. https://doi.org/10.1037/0003-066X.61.8.774.

and trauma, encourages moral behavior, and can help build social bonds.

Thus, Called to Care providers should always be grateful for opportunities to positively affect our patients' lives. It's what we were called to do.[100]

How You Can Start a Simple Gratitude Practice

Every February 18th, the positive psychology academic community encourages an exercise in honor of one of its founders, Christopher Peterson. Alongside Martin Seligman and Mihaly Csikszentmihalyi, they are considered the driving forces behind this modern field. Peterson's extensive contributions to positive psychology include being author and co-author of more than 350 scholarly publications and books, including *A Primer in Positive Psychology, Character Strengths and Virtues* and *Pursuing the Good Life: 100 Reflections on Positive Psychology.* He is known for his mantra "other people matter" and his contributions to authoring, validating, and promoting positive psychology interventions, including most notably, gratitude. This exercise involves writing a handwritten letter to a person you are particularly grateful to have in your life. It is helpful to be detailed and express all of the wonderful qualities about this person and how they have personally affected

---

100 Lyubomirsky, Sonja. *The How of Happiness: A New Approach to Getting the Life You Want.* New York: Penguin Press, 2007.

your life for the better. It is highly recommended to personally deliver this message.

Best Practices

Besides the classic blessings exercise and gratitude letter, there are a ton of others that have been published. In our experience, the following have significant benefits.

Journaling

In his book *Thanks*, Dr. Robert Emmons details a study in which one group of subjects were told to write five things they were grateful for each week, while another group was told to write five things they were displeased about each week. After ten weeks, the results revealed that those who wrote about gratitude were 25 percent happier than the other group and the control group. Additionally, they reported more exercise and fewer health complaints than the other groups. While writing about gratitude in general can be beneficial, research also shows that the more specific you are about what you are grateful for, the more beneficial your gratitude journaling will be. A study from the University of Southern California backs up this research. In their study, the researchers found that test subjects who wrote five sentences about one thing they were grateful for were happier and more energetic compared to test subjects who were asked to write about just one sentence about five things they were grateful for over the course of ten weeks.[101] So when you're journaling, make sure to be specific! Instead of saying you're grateful for your spouse, for example, go into detail about why you are grateful for them, citing specific personality traits, experiences, and things they have done for you in the past.

Write "Thank You" Notes

In his book *365 Thank Yous: The Year a Simple Act of Daily Gratitude Changed My Life*, John Kralik explains how writing one thank-you note each day for 365 consecutive days transformed his life. John notes starting this exercise with everyone that gave him a Christmas gift, and then expanding to coworkers, then to other people he interacted with, such as a barista that greeted him by name at his local Starbucks. From this experience, John realized that writing the thank-you notes helped him focus on little things he had been taking for granted and to be more positive about the bad things in his life. After his 365-day exercise was over, he noticed that his life had changed significantly. He lost weight, his failing business was prospering, and his relationships with family and friends had improved.

---

101 Emmons, Robert A. *Gratitude Works! A 21-Day Program for Creating Emotional Prosperity*. San Francisco, CA: Jossey-Bass, 2013.

Meditate with Gratitude

Gratitude expression and meditation are two wellness practices that can significantly increase your happiness. Combining them into one meditation experience can make your results even more significant. Instead of keeping your mind clear like you would with typical meditation, gratitude meditation involves concentrating and reflecting on being grateful for everything in your life—both the bad and the good. You can meditate on the happiness the good things in your life bring, as well as recognize the opportunities for growth the seemingly bad things in life can bring about.

Daily App

There are tons of apps for mobile devices that enhance habits and rituals. These apps allow you to customize categories and then evaluate quickly whether or not you performed them at whatever interval of time you determine. I suggest the gratitude category be a question—what are you grateful for today? This compels one to reflect and name something. For more impact, you can fill in why you are grateful for that one thing today.

For more resources on this topic, visit CalledtoCarebook. com.

CHAPTER TEN

HOW TO BEGIN MAKING EMPATHY A DAILY PRACTICE

"Empathy is seeing with the eyes of another, listening with the ears of another and feeling with the heart of another."

—ALFRED ADLER

The Extinction of Empathy

Many patients face impediments in healthcare today—the dearth of primary care physicians, limitations imposed by health insurance plans, and exceedingly long wait times to see certain doctors. However, a greater focus on empathy can yield a myriad of benefits for patients, even in these challenging times. Picture friendly and supportive staff members, shorter wait times, quality reading material, games and toys for children, and ancillary education.

Furthermore, through our Called to Care initiative, which originally focused on physical therapists, we have demonstrated empirically that you can shift providers' behaviors in ways that enhance compassion, kindness, positivity, and empathy toward patients and thereby significantly enhancing patients' experiences in a number of ways. In fact, it is my contention that care excellence, coupled with clinical and service excellence, are the pillars necessary for creating the best clinical outcomes. "Care excellence" includes positivity, compassion, shaping patient expectations, and empathy.

Within a clinical context, empathy is a predominantly cognitive (versus emotional) attribute that involves an understanding (versus a feeling) of experiences, concerns, and perspectives of the patient, combined with a capacity to communicate this understanding.[102] In fact, as previously noted, a lack of empathy is believed to contribute to the burnout or attrition rates of healthcare providers, particularly those who work with traumatized clients; thus, it was surprising to discover that mental health workers

---

102 Hojat, Mohammadreza. *Empathy in Patient Care: Antecedents, Development, Measurement, and Outcomes.* New York: Springer Science & Business Media, 2007.

with "exquisite empathy"[103] were found to be invigorated (versus depleted) by their intimate professional connections with traumatized clients (and were thus protected against compassion fatigue and burnout).

When I began this journey, it was surprising to me to learn that empathy, when viewed as a measured strength from Gallup's StrengthsFinder, is not as prevalent in healthcare as I had anticipated. In fact, our extensive internal studies most frequently place empathy in the bottom five of thirty-four strengths measured. Perhaps the definition of empathy from StrengthsFinder ("the empathy theme can sense the feelings of other people by imagining themselves in others' lives or situations") is not encompassing enough to be transported into a healthcare environment.[104]

As previously noted from the study of *Wit* and the "Don Quixote Effect," despite the importance of the humanities and arts in enhancing empathy, many medical schools and most physical therapy programs have not incorporated these subjects in their curricula; in fact, it has been reported that only a third of all the medical schools in the United

103 Harrison, Richard L., and Westwood, Marvin J. "Preventing Vicarious Traumatization of Mental Health Therapists: Identifying Protective Practices." *Psychotherapy: Theory, Research, Practice, Training* 46, no. 2 (2009): 203-19. https://doi.org/10.1037/a0016081.

104 Rath, Tom, and Conchie, Barry. *Strengths Based Leadership: Great Leaders, Teams, and Why People Follow.* New York: Gallup Press, 2009.

States had incorporated literature into their curricula as of the mid-1990s.[105,106,107]

Furthermore, regardless of the degree of empathy, many licensed medical providers are at risk of losing their empathic skills the longer they stay in practice; this may be considered part of the dehumanization process in an age and culture with too much focus on acquisition and status versus values, and healthcare environments facing daunting regulations and compliance pressures. Relatedly, in chapter 8, we identified this dehumanization process is often triggered in part by a disproportionate exposure to a negative environment or excessive patient care hours resulting in *calcification* or becoming numb to human connections and emotions. While calcification is not synonymous with lack of empathy, it is best likened as a temporary loss of empathy. Understanding how the process evolves in a natural or due course of a workday is a key measure of using techniques that decalcify or rehumanize.

Thus, healthcare practitioners who are part of the Called to Care initiative receive empathy training in addition to

---

105 Charon, R., Banks, J.T., Connelly, J.E., Hawkins, A.H., Hunter, K.M., Jones, A.H., Montello, M., and Poirer, S. "Literature and Medicine: Contributions to Clinical Practice." *Annals of Internal Medicine* 122, no. 8 (1995): 599–606. https://doi.org/10.7326/0003-4819-122-8-199504150-00008.

106 Jones, Anne Hudson. "Literature and Medicine: Narrative Ethics." *The Lancet* 349, no. 9060 (1997): 1243–46. https://doi.org/10.1016/s0140-6736(97)03395-3.

107 Hunter, K.M., Charon, R., and Coulehan, J.L. "The Study of Literature in Medical Education." *Academic Medicine* 70, no. 9 (1995): 787–94.

understanding the need for heightened sensitivity to the naturally occurring dehumanization process. We feel that empathy is a strategic competitive advantage that differentiates practitioners in the evolving healthcare-delivery landscape, one that not only emphasizes patient-centric focus, but lives it. To those that question the impact of empathy on clinical outcomes, Rakel, Barrett, Zhang, et al. (2011) did an ingenious study on 719 patients who presented with symptoms of the common cold. Those who were treated with an "enhanced encounter" designed as one in which practitioners were taught and emphasized empathy, were rated as perfect on patient-measured instruments as well as had decreased severity, duration, and confirmed reduction in neutrophils versus those who were in a control group and a standard encounter.[108]

Mindfulness as an Empathy Builder

An important tool for cultivating empathy in today's challenging healthcare environment is mindfulness. Perhaps more than any other body of research, we have more evidence on mindfulness and its effect than on any other current area of scientific thinking. Mindfulness is nonjudgmental awareness coupled with collaboration and a sense of humility. Literally defined, it is paying attention in

---

108 Rakel, David, Barrett, Bruce, Zhang, Zhengjun, Hoeft, Theresa, Chewning, Betty, Marchand, Lucille, and Scheder, Jo. "Perception of Empathy in the Therapeutic Encounter: Effects on the Common Cold." *Patient Education and Counseling* 85, no. 3 (2011): 390–97. https://doi.org/10.1016/j.pec.2011.01.009.

a particular way, on purpose, to the present moment, and without judgment. Mindfulness is the ability to focus at the moment on what is important—in this case, the patient in front of you—or perhaps even yourself.

Of course, mindlessness is commonly a byproduct of multitasking, or trying to do too many "too manys" at one time. Multitasking is viewed as a skill. Unfortunately, research tells us that we can't really multitask—that we are simply shifting from one task to another and both tasks get shortchanged in the process. Unlike skill building, the more we practice multitasking, the worse we get at it.

Medical providers are put in the position to multitask far too often, such as focusing on an electronic medical record while your patient is telling you something important about his or her condition or history. Fortunately, it takes just eight minutes of training, consisting of paying attention in a particular way, on purpose, in the present moment, and nonjudgmentally, which is the definition crafted by Jon Kabat-Zinn, noted author and mindfulness-based stress-reduction founder. This state particularly includes focused breathing and reaps incredible benefits in multiple ways.

Another antidote for mind-wandering is meta-awareness (i.e., attention to attention itself); this is the ability to notice that you are not noticing what you should be focusing on and thus correcting it by refocusing. Mindfulness can make this critical muscle stronger.

Mindfulness training really does five things:

1. It decreases mind-wandering.
2. It shifts attention quickly (i.e., it allows you to shift attention "in the zone" quickly).
3. It allows you to focus longer, which is a critical skill and deliberate practice.
4. It allows you to observe your own mental processes rather than be swept away by them.
5. It provides an enhancement of executive function. It is a time gap between impulse and action.

The best part of mindfulness training? It is free, straightforward, and proven. Mindfulness has many benefits, and the Called to Care providers adopt a steady and consistent practice. Fortunately, many apps, tutors, and ubiquity of mindfulness opportunities make an ongoing practice easier to maintain.

Other Subtle Ways to Build Empathy

Other tools to make part of your daily practice include pause breaks, an on-purpose, temporary, intentional break that enables active disengagement. Pause breaks are personal. For some, it is a few mindfulness breaths; for others, it is simply a meditation, prayer, silence, distraction, or other techniques known as "brain hacks." For me, my personal pause break routine was having a *USA Today* crossword puzzle or sudoku handy as my intention was to solve it between patients. Pause breaks allow feelings, emotions, and blind spots to evolve and play out or dissipate. Upon completion, you can come back to your patient stronger and more empathetic without being blinded by bias, fatigue, or calcification.

Also, touch seems to impart a subliminal sense of caring and connection.[109] Interestingly, a very light touch has even been found to increase the number of people who agree to sign a petition, the chances that a college student will risk embarrassment by going to the blackboard in a statistics class, the proportion of busy passersby in a mall who will take a ten-minute survey, and the percentage of shoppers in a supermarket who purchased food that they had sampled.

Of course, some people might be skeptical of this; after all, some of us recoil when a stranger touches us, and it is possible that some of the subjects in the studies did. However, these reactions were far outweighed by the reactions of those who reacted positively. Surprisingly, in studies in which the touched person was later debriefed about the

---

109 Willis, Frank N., and Hamm, Helen K. "The Use of Interpersonal Touch in Securing Compliance." *Journal of Nonverbal Behavior* 5, no. 1 (1980): 49–55. https://doi.org/10.1007/bf00987054.

experience, typically less than one-third of the subjects were even aware that they had been touched.

For years, I have taught our physical therapists that our differentiation is based on being a "hands-on" profession. We are one of the few providers that through physical examination, manual therapy, and a variety of interventions that physically "touch" patients, and this is a critical piece of connecting as well. My encouragement for all providers is to be "hands-on" in a professional, caring way. Far too many of our patients tell us that their [choose any medical provider] simply took diagnostic tests and gave out prescriptions without ever examining or touching them. Called to Care providers never underestimate this important piece of connection.

CONCLUSION

To summarize, some of the best healthcare practitioners today are attempting to utilize heart and mind to optimize patient outcomes. They realize their own baggage, often in the form of cognitive biases, and know they have to work on these cognitive abilities just as much as their manual skills. They learn that becoming nonjudgmental and overcoming fast-brain biases is a more difficult task than anything else and it takes desire, practice, feedback, and training.

The best Called to Care providers understand that they are being judged on a continuum of warm, friendly, smart competence and that they need to apply these factors to every patient and see things from his or her perspective. The purpose of this book is to renew efforts to bring humanity back to healthcare. We have plenty of evidence but not enough care in my view. Furthermore, it is time to bring the evidence of care and compassion to the forefront of healthcare.

Many of the evidence-based information presented are direct interventions to patients. For example, using high-quality connections, broaden-and-build positivity, goal setting, active constructive communication, effective use of the "peak-end" rule, empathy, compassion, and the dramatic impact of influencing placebo and mitigating nocebo. Other interventions, including gratitude, identifying "triggers" of calcification, and having a mindfulness practice are for the provider. We cannot effectively provide healthcare if, as providers, we aren't engaging in our own health, physical as well as mental.

We make special emphasis on empathy because it is a far deeper multidimensional construct than the reflexive "walk in the moccasins" approach we have been led to believe. Empathy is "thinking," "feeling," and "action" oriented in an environment of nonjudgment. Neuroscientists have identified the empathy center of anterior insular cortex but also the frontal, somatosensory cortex, and the amygdala. I have participated in the debate about empathy with one solid group of academics entrenched in the position that it is not empathy that we want as medical providers but compassion. Their argument in part is that empathy can be personalized to our own detriment. I disagree based on my perspective that empathy must be understood at four distinct levels and the realization that the most empathetic professionals have the longest staying power as medical professionals. It is my opinion that they also get the best results for their patients.

This is not to suggest that I am not a fan of compassion. Compassion, or the ability to see a person potentially as yourself, is one of the major constructs of empathy and is thus a skill. Scientists have identified the right temporo-parietal junction (RTPJ), whose only function is to see others' perspectives. Every time you put yourself in another's shoes, it lights up. Thus, compassion is a shared connection with others or literally interpreted means suffering with one another. Both empathy and compassion are about shared experiences. It is our skill or ability to tap into our own experiences in order to connect with an experience someone is relating to us. Compassion is the willingness to be open to this process. If compassion is more intuitive, teachable, and refining as a skill than empathy then please feel free to emphasize it versus empathy. In our experience, we find teaching empathy is scalable and necessary (please visit CalledtoCarebook. com for a presentation on "10 Things You Need to Know about Empathy"). We also have to acknowledge that the empathy "muscle" needs replenishment. Significant research including students in physical therapy departing for their final internships has shown that empathy can be lost but then regained but it takes an intentional effort, both personally and organizationally, to keep it top of mind.

Results of our internal studies using the Consultation and Relational Empathy (CARE) instrument demonstrate that if you keep providers accountable to patient perspectives and empathy with frequent feedback from this validated instrument that providers do, in fact, rise to the occasion and maintain a patient-centric approach including listening, positivity, understanding, consideration of the whole person, and explaining. In our view, it is our organization's responsibility to hold our entire team, from the front desk to the billing department, to a high level of accountability, and without objective surveys, deliberate feedback, and ongoing training, our efforts would be just a short-term initiative with little long-standing sustainability.

I am fond of telling our team that common sense is not common practice and it is our imperative to make common sense common practice. Most of the evidence-based transportable positive psychological interventions are just that—common sense. My sincere encouragement and hope is that you, too, will make these common practices. Our healthcare system desperately needs it.

Here's to bringing humanity back to healthcare.

APPENDIX A

ROLLING OUT *CALLED TO CARE* THROUGH APPRECIATIVE INQUIRY

A Prescription for Managing the Ills of Modern-Day Healthcare

"We live in the world our questions create."

—DAVID COOPERRIDER

Many of us have witnessed on a daily basis that the healthcare industry is full of heroes who have dedicated their careers to restoring health.[110] Thus, it is very fortunate that even though we are all under tremendous pressure in these uncertain times, there are strategies to help us navigate and routines we can begin to utilize to transform our

---

110 May, Natalie, Becker, Daniel M., and Frankel, Richard M. *Appreciative Inquiry in Healthcare: Positive Questions to Bring out the Best.* Brunswick, OH: Crown Custom Publishing, Inc., 2011.

organizations and even our careers. As we begin to bring this all together, I would like to take a look at one final technique, one that is recommended for an intentional rollout of *Called to Care*: Appreciative Inquiry (AI).

AI is a change paradigm grounded in strengths-oriented innovation and is focused on looking for the best in people and organizations (i.e., the "positive core").[111] The kind of practical questions that AI promotes can transform conversations and promote positivity and life-affirming directions. AI begins by formulating the change agenda: that is, determining what the objective of the process should be.[112] This should be positive, visionary, and transformational—just what healthcare needs.

The AI process generally consists of four stages, called the 4D model:

1. Discovery—reflections and discussions focusing on what is best about the object of inquiry
2. Dream—imagining the objective at its best and synthesizing a shared vision and common aspirations
3. Design—generating concrete proposals for how the dream might look

---

111 Cooperrider, David L., Stavros, Jacqueline M., and Whitney, Diana. *Appreciative Inquiry Handbook: for Leaders of Change*, 2nd ed. San Francisco, CA: Berrett-Koehler Publishers, 2008.

112 Cooperrider, David L., Stavros, Jacqueline M., and Whitney, Diana. *Appreciative Inquiry Handbook: for Leaders of Change*, 2nd ed. San Francisco, CA: Berrett-Koehler Publishers, 2008.

4. Destiny—making it happen[113,114,115]

AI is a highly effective method for solving organizational issues and one we have utilized at Confluent Health. Through our initiative, *Called to Care*, we hosted our first AI summit for physical therapists on January 29, 2013. Our key question was, "What do you want to create?" We focused specifically on our profession's strengths—what we are doing well—and on the promising future of healthcare organizations that focus on compassionate, kind, and positive care. Our plan was to facilitate change via a collaborative learning management platform using positive psychology principles.

We used AI, in part, to obtain buy-in so that staff would embrace this positive, experiential method and feel liberated by it. We defined our vision by sharing positive inquiry stories. These included imagining the ideal clinical environment and learning from experiences when we were fully listening to, and connecting with, our patients. Our original summit was attended by physical therapists with differing levels of experience. Attendees included recent graduates,

113 Bushe, G.R. "Appreciative Inquiry: Theory and Critique." In *The Routledge Companion to Organizational Change*, edited by D. Boje, B. Burnes, and J. Hassard, 87-103. Oxford, UK: Routledge, 2011.

114 Cooperrider, David L., Stavros, Jacqueline M., and Whitney, Diana. *Appreciative Inquiry Handbook: for Leaders of Change*, 2nd ed. San Francisco, CA: Berrett-Koehler Publishers, 2008.

115 Whitney, Diana, and Trosten-Bloom, Amanda. *The Power of Appreciative Inquiry a Practical Guide to Positive Change*, 2nd ed. San Francisco, CA: Berrett-Koehler Publishers, Inc., 2010.

mid-career and seasoned professionals, interns, residents, and students. The breadth and depth of this community experience was a tremendous asset. By strategically coupling therapists for the paired interviews and placing them in small groups, the summit proved to be highly informative.

At the conclusion of our AI Summit, a thirty-minute, high-level overview was presented with evidence-based Called to Care materials for clinical integration, essentially a concise version of each of the chapters of this book. This was meant to further curiosity and give direction to the learning management system (LMS) that we utilize for deeper learning and further collaboration amongst participants, the deep dive of these same chapters. The topics, or the chapters of this book, were chosen for their relevance, degree of supporting evidence, ease of integration, and ability to enhance well-being among clinicians as well as patients. In this context, each topic began with a professionally recorded and edited video lecture. Additional resources included publicly available videos, documents, websites, and a discussion board to encourage collaboration among participants and the integration of materials into clinical practice. The momentum of the Called to Care initiative was maintained in various ways (e.g., results reports, intercompany newsletters highlighting superstar results, and frequent additions of resources and videos). We now offer this "deep dive" through Evidence in Motion at evidenceinmotion.com/course/online-called-to-care.

For the most part, our AI summits have focused on AI's *discovery* and *dream* components, the key constructs as defined by the developer, David Cooperrider. The *discovery* phase (appreciating the best of what is) helps us to identify the key strengths and assets of our industry and profession. Questions explore the joy and meaning of physical therapy, as well as issues pertaining to connecting (and listening) to patients. The *dream* (or imagining) stage has focused on what could be considered relevant to kind, compassionate, and positive care. Participants have provided their best input as they have begun to feel that they are part of something larger. They have shared emotionally engaging stories about patient care; the experience of contributing to this initiative provided momentum, enabled cultural change, and solidified team commitment.

Most importantly, AI can be implemented for different change objectives and different groups: from individuals, to small groups, to organizations, to the world.[116,117,118] AI summits have been used effectively by companies and communities to generate transformational change, and in particular for "crafting inspiring and generative visions

116 Bushe, G.R. "Appreciative Inquiry: Theory and Critique." In *The Routledge Companion to Organizational Change*, edited by D. Boje, B. Burnes, and J. Hassard, 87-103. Oxford, UK: Routledge, 2011.

117 Cooperrider, David L., Stavros, Jacqueline M., and Whitney, Diana. *Appreciative Inquiry Handbook: for Leaders of Change*, 2nd ed. San Francisco, CA: Berrett-Koehler Publishers, 2008.

118 Whitney, Diana, and Trosten-Bloom, Amanda. *The Power of Appreciative Inquiry a Practical Guide to Positive Change*, 2nd ed. San Francisco, CA: Berrett-Koehler Publishers, Inc., 2010.

of the future" and "forging mergers, alliances, and partnerships,"[119] both of which fit the goals and objectives of Called to Care. We strongly suggest AI as the platform for rolling out *Called to Care* but want to make sure to emphasize that AI can be utilized for deploying many monumental organizational initiatives.

Step-by-Step AI for Organizations and Summits

The following provides a step-by-step guide to help you utilize AI tools in group settings as a precursor to *Called to Care* implementation or other effort focused on bringing empathy, humanization, or renewed patient-centric care to your setting. This process is designed to highlight your organizational strengths and positive situations via a series of questions and discussions. These exercises should be completed in a comfortable group setting, and it is best for the entire organization to participate together.

Opening Inquiry

In your group setting, ask group members to break off into pairs and talk about the following discussion question. Ask one person to share his or her thoughts for fifteen minutes, while the second person listens and takes brief notes. Then

---

119 Whitney, Diana, and Trosten-Bloom, Amanda. *The Power of Appreciative Inquiry a Practical Guide to Positive Change*, 2nd ed. San Francisco, CA: Berrett-Koehler Publishers, Inc., 2010.

have the pair switch roles and repeat the process for fifteen minutes.

Share, or talk about, a time when the pieces came together, and you and your team delivered exceptional care to a patient.

Once this exercise is complete, bring group members back together and ask the pairs to share. Have each person share his or her partner's story—not his or her own. Make sure to encourage sharing via positive comments from meeting leaders.

Paired Conversation Interview

Share the following statements with the entire group:

"Humane-oriented leadership emphasizes being supportive, considerate, compassionate, and generous. This type of leadership includes modesty and sensitivity to other people."

—PETER G. NORTHOUSE, *LEADERSHIP: THEORY AND PRACTICE*

"Everyone is a leader because everyone influences someone."

—JOHN MAXWELL

Ask the group to again break off into pairs, either the same pairs as before or different ones. Once the group members have broken off into pairs, ask them to consider and discuss the following questions. They should be prepared to share their stories.

Elaborate on the time that the pieces came together, and you and your team delivered exceptional care to a patient:

- When and where did it happen?
- Describe what happened and how you contributed.
- What made this experience a high point for you?
- What were the challenges—and, more importantly, how were they overcome?

Drawing on this story and others like it, what are your best qualities or strengths? Think of others who know and work with you: what would they say are your three best qualities or strengths?

After approximately twenty to thirty minutes of discussion time, bring the group back together, and ask for volunteers to share some of their stories. Make sure to encourage sharing via positive comments from meeting leaders.

Table Discussion

Now form groups of four to six people. You should provide the following instructions to each group:

1. A facilitator, a timekeeper, a recorder, and a reporter should be selected within your group.
2. The facilitator should keep the group moving through the exercises noted below.
3. The timekeeper aids the facilitator by ensuring that the group is moving through the exercises with enough time to complete all assigned tasks within the allotted time.
4. The recorder will document group discussions on a flip-chart, computer, or on paper.

Once the groups have selected their facilitator, timekeeper, recorder, and reporter, assign one of the following interview questions to each group. Each group should have a different question. (If you have more than seven groups, you can reassign questions; if you have fewer than seven groups, pick the questions you prefer but do not assign the same questions to multiple groups.)

Interview Questions:

1. Talk about a time when you had a peak experience in compassionate caring.
2. When have you felt most connected to your patient?
3. Describe a time when you really listened and it made a big difference.
4. Talk about the last time a patient thanked you for listening. What did you do or say that allowed the patient

(or his or her family) to ask the right questions at the right time?

5. Describe a time when you were able to make time stand still, forget about other obligations, and be completely in the moment.

6. What would a new patient's ideal first visit to your clinic look like?

7. What were your hopes and aspirations when you chose healthcare as a profession?

8. What provides you with the greatest joy and meaning in your work?

9. What do you like the most about being a healthcare provider with our company?

Next, ask the groups to complete the following exercises:

1. Go around the table and introduce your paired conversation partner (from the previous exercise). Share a couple of highlights from your previous discussion—things from your partner's responses that stood out most to you.

2. Use the remaining time to deeply discuss the interview question assigned to you. Share your stories and observations, ask for group members' input, and listen for patterns or themes.

3. Following this exercise, the reporter will be asked to share themes and patterns from each group's discussion with the overall group.

After about thirty to forty minutes of discussion time, bring the group back together and ask for volunteers to share some of their stories. These stories will likely elicit many emotions and be important to those sharing them. Make sure to encourage sharing with positive comments from the meeting leaders.

For healthcare professionals, the AI process may be initiated by reflecting on your career at a time when kindness, compassion, empathy, and a sense of calling were unquestionably demonstrated. To explore this, it is advisable to write about a time involving a peak experience in compassionate caring while considering such questions as:

- What provides you with the greatest joy and meaning in your work?
- What were your hopes and aspirations when you chose this line of work?
- What would a new patient's first visit to your place of business ideally look like?

Thus, AI may also be used by individuals; it is a method of problem-solving that we use often here at Confluent Health. As you address associated professional issues, please always remember to emphasize the importance of making your patients and coworkers feel important. Patients, in particular, need to feel like they are a priority—particularly when they visit your clinic.

Step-by-Step AI for Individuals

Reflect on your career and remember moments of kindness, compassion, empathy, and your sense of calling to your profession via the following step-by-step guide to *Appreciative Inquiry for Individuals*. The following steps will help you learn from others in the healthcare industry, provide an outlet for your own thinking, and enable you to reflect on personal experiences.

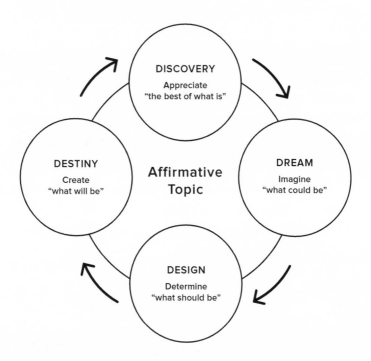

Design

Write about a time when you had a peak experience in compassionate caring. When did you feel most connected to your patient? Examples from other healthcare professionals are provided below.

....

....

....

Peak Experience Examples

- Providing education to patients (because they typically don't get that with all healthcare professionals)
- Standing up for a patient with post-traumatic stress disorder (e.g., going above and beyond to make the patient feel as comfortable as possible)
- Showing compassion and caring (e.g., asking about the patient's family and/or personal life)
- Attending funerals
- Asking about a new baby

Also:

- Feel out different personality types and adapt and react accordingly
- Be able to joke with/tease patients as a means of connecting (since humor and play are part of compassionate care)

Consider when you feel most connected with your patients:

- When you joke around with them, you treat them as a friend or family member and not as "Mrs. Jones's knees."
- When the patient starts asking you about you, a two-way connection is occurring.

Discovery

What provides you with the greatest joy and meaning in your work? (Examples from other healthcare professionals are provided below.)

....

....

....

Example:

- When we get patients who are truly at the end of their rope (after having been everywhere)—and then we find the answer, help them, and see that:
  - They are happy to have someone listen.
  - We give them hope.
  - We get them back to their professions/hobbies/families.
  - We give them their lives back.

Even when patients don't get the recovery they were seeking, they at least often have the glimmer of hope that they can get there. Additionally, it can be rewarding when we see other healthcare professionals getting better at their jobs; this alone can be inspiring.

Dreaming

What were your hopes and aspirations when you chose healthcare as a profession? (Examples from other healthcare professionals are provided below.)

....

....

....

Examples:

- Finding a job that would make an impact and provide a purpose
- Wanting to work with people
- Job security
- Flexibility
- Working with a variety of patients in a variety of settings
- Wanting to hear patient stories
- Wanting to help people

- Making a difference in the lives of coworkers
- Autonomy

It's important to remember that most healthcare professionals go into this field because it's a calling, so it's okay to dream big!

Destiny

Ideally, what would a new patient's first visit to your organization look like? (Examples from other healthcare professionals are provided below.)

....

....

....

Examples:

- A patient's first impression of your practice is often your building, so you should consider offering:
  - A presentable entryway
  - A good, clean environment
  - Carefully maintained landscaping
  - A friendly greeting at the front desk

Remember that if anything around your office seems "off," you may leave your patients wondering what kind of care they are going to get. Thus, your attention to detail should include your work directly with your patients, the time you take to answer questions, and your ability to clarify forms and benefits. Clinicians should greet patients on time and remember to:

- Introduce themselves
- Shake hands
- Call patients by name
- Chat with patients while walking to treatment rooms
- Listen to patients
- Provide appropriate treatments
- Let patients know what to expect in terms of the process, timeline, and expected outcomes
- Answer questions
- Lead patients to the front desk
- Offer a number to call at any time
- Stay at the front desk to help patients schedule upcoming visits

APPENDIX B

CALLED TO CARE VALIDATED

The Called to Care program used the validated Consultation and Relational Empathy (CARE) measure to monitor original program results, which incorporated the key constructs of positive psychology that are part of the curriculum, including empathy, quality connections, and positivity.[120] CARE also has a normative database that allows comparison of our results with various databases, notably a dataset of 62,357 questionnaires from 1,520 different professionals, including physiotherapists (the British term for "physical therapist") from the UK. Over 13,000 new patients of trained physical therapists from five physical therapy clinics

---

120 Mercer, S. W. "The Consultation and Relational Empathy (CARE) Measure: Development and Preliminary Validation and Reliability of an Empathy-Based Consultation Process Measure." *Family Practice* 21, no. 6 (2004): 699-705. https://doi.org/10.1093/fampra/cmh621.

in Texas were given a confidential space and mobile platform to enter their responses to the ten questions after their initial visit (Exhibit 1). The questions reflect the following on a five-part Likert scale, from fair to excellent.

How was the physical therapist at:

1. Making you feel at ease
2. Letting you tell your story
3. Really listening
4. Being interested in you as a whole person
5. Fully understanding your concerns
6. Showing care and compassion
7. Being positive
8. Explaining things clearly
9. Helping you take control
10. Making a plan of action with you

The following table compares scores from the normative database to the combined scores of five physical therapy clinics:

	BASELINE NORMATIVE AVERAGES	CALLED TO CARE THERAPISTS AVERAGES
Q1: EASE	4.618	4.843
Q2: STORY	4.526	4.851
Q3: LISTEN	4.572	4.849
Q4: WHOLE PERSON	4.493	4.778
Q5: UNDERSTANDING	4.521	4.844
Q6: CARE	4.557	4.833
Q7: POSITIVE	4.561	4.855
Q8: EXPLAINING	4.611	4.843
Q9: CONTROL	4.058	4.710
Q10: ACTION	4.532	4.780
AVERAGE OF ALL QUESTIONS	4.505	4.819
MEDIAN	4.544	4.843
MODE	NA	4.843
FULL SCORE	45.4838	48.186
NUMBER OF RESPONSES	6943	1314

A two-tailed t-test was calculated (p-value = .0001, 95 percent confidence interval), which demonstrated significant differences on every question and the overall full score. The data strongly suggest that the impact of training physical therapists produces a shift in their behavior, which influences patients' reports of therapists' empathy, listening, positivity, and other related measures.

I acknowledge that this program is not based on direct research; however, its design is built on theoretical and empirical foundations. While we are certain that the normative database of medical providers has not been through Called to Care, we cannot attest that they have not had any training in empathy or on topics related to positive psychology. We have also assumed that Called to Care therapists have completed all components of this training, but we cannot verify this entirely. An additional limitation would include the lack of a control group of physical therapists in the United States that have not been through training. Nonetheless, each question within the CARE measure (and the overall score) shows a statistically significant difference between Called to Care physical therapy participants and the normative database, indicating the potential that this theoretically and empirically based application of positive psychology is having significant effects on the patient–provider care experience.

Future Endeavors for Called to Care

The CARE measure has demonstrated that training and implementation of Called to Care have resulted in statistically significantly higher scores than a normative database across all intervention issues, including empathy, care and compassion, listening, positivity, clear explanation, and allowing patients to tell their story. However, we also plan to assess clinical, workforce, and financial outcomes to see if the program has had an effect. We know from internal studies that we did, after the implementation of Called to Care, following correlation with third-party clinical outcomes tracking and third-party collection of patient loyalty scores, that the best clinical outcomes were facilitated by Called to Care physical therapists with the highest CARE measures. From a clinical standpoint, CARE measures might be an easy proxy for functional outcomes. In terms of workforce outcomes, we are exploring the relationship with therapist engagement before and after Called to Care using the standardized Gallup engagement survey we have been using for years. Our initial analysis is promising, and we believe, given the high engagement scores and their increase over pre-Called to Care, that this might be a good proxy for therapists and their calling. Lastly, we are analyzing different business metrics (e.g., visits per patient, no show/cancellation rates, patient retention, and word-of-mouth referrals) in order to make a convincing case that this program also can be justified purely from a financial investment.

Through *Called to Care* and related initiatives, I believe that we will add significantly to positive health, resulting in kinder, more compassionate care, better outcomes, a reinvigoration to professional calling, and a clear distinction from mainstream healthcare. More importantly, it will be fully embraced by patients and be seen as necessary and refreshing.

APPENDIX C

CHECKLIST FOR CALLED TO CARE SKILLS

To ensure success when implementing Called to Care, it is critical to integrate three key ingredients:

1. A skills checklist
2. Systems approach
3. Deliberate practice

In managing healthcare providers of varying types, we have created or overseen a variety of skills checklists, and we recommend this approach for Called to Care. As an example, the military identified more than one hundred skills and tasks that are required for a combat medic to become efficient in providing high-quality combat casualty care.

These skills are identified and described in objective detail, and instructors are provided resources and training tools. A competency checklist is also created, and after thorough and consistent training, assessments are done on each medic to ensure they have been properly trained and can perform these critical tasks. Working with several of our academic partners, we have used this same approach to teach physical therapists evidence-based, hands-on interventions as well as examination and patient interviewing techniques. Each provider is given a mentor whose duties include holding the provider accountable for implementing these skills.

In our experience, implementing cognitive or emotional intelligence skills, like rehumanization or "soft" skills for Called to Care providers, is challenging. The typical experience for medical providers is that hands-on or fine motor skills are much more emphasized in medical training through mentoring, lab sessions, ongoing practice, replication, simulation, and testing. While it is daunting, the best way to integrate, ensure, and hold providers accountable for the development of their soft skills is by having a skills checklist that holds them to the same standards of rigor as they experience with the learning of hands-on skills. To that end, we have taken a systems approach that incorporates a comprehensive methodology around implementation. The components of this systems approach are "define it," "teach it," "live it," "monitor it," "reward it," "improve it," "redefine it," and start over, as depicted:

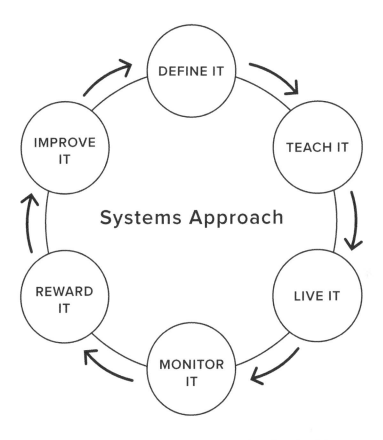

This approach provides ongoing renewal and replenishment of skills and competencies, and it avoids a decline in skills despite more years of experience. Extensive research in a wide range of fields shows many people do not get better at skills no matter how many years they spend practicing. We refer to this phenomenon as "not fourteen years of experience but one year of experience repeated fourteen times." As it turns out, this does not just happen in healthcare, but it also occurs in auditors, psychologists, stockbrokers, parole officers, and college admissions specialists. At times, people get worse with experience, including some physicians, who score lower on medical knowledge tests than less-experienced physicians and some general physicians who become less-skilled over time at diagnosing heart sounds and radiographs.[121]

Anders Ericsson, the Florida State University psychologist credited with the "10,000-hour rule," has identified that the main predictor of success is deliberate practice. This is defined as persistent training that requires full concentration in chunks of focused time, often guided by a skilled expert, mentor, or coach. This type of practice is not about clocking hours; it is the way the practice is done that makes the biggest difference. As a general rule, our amount of productive failure helps determine our ultimate success. Key components of the deliberate practice approach require a motivation to attend to the task, demonstrated improvement in performance, immediate and informative feedback, and an ability to repeatedly perform the same or similar tasks. Such intentionality is necessary for hands-on, cognitive, and emotional regulation skills.[122]

To that end, we have created this checklist for Called to

---

121 Ericsson, K. A., Krampe, R. T., and Tesch-Römer, C. "The Role of Deliberate Practice in the Acquisition of Expert Performance." *Psychological Review* 100, no. 3 (1993): 363–406. https://doi.org/10.1037/0033-295x.100.3.363.

122 Ericsson, K. A. "Deliberate Practice and Acquisition of Expert Performance: A General Overview." *Academic Emergency Medicine* 15, no. 11 (2008): 988–94. https://doi.org/10.1111/j.1553-2712.2008.00227.x.

Care skills, so that you can approach the necessary skills for success with deliberation and intention. For each of the *Called to Care* chapters, we have identified intervention(s), some points to consider, some reminders, and in some cases further examples. What follows is our skills checklist for the Called to Care provider.

Chapter One—High-Quality Connections and Empathy

Points and reminders:

- The quality of high-quality connection is marked by three subjective experiences: vitality, positive, and mutuality.
- If a feeling is unshared, then it is sympathy: "I see the emotion but have a different emotion."
- Empathy is marked by four very distinct concepts:
  - Cognitive: also known as perspective-taking, i.e., "walking in your shoes"
  - Emotional: I mirror or "feel" the shared emotion and legitimize it.
  - Prosocial concern: I am motivated to help and to problem solve.
  - All under the atmosphere of nonjudgment

Chapter Two—Broaden-and-Build

A few talking points listed as a reminder:

- The broaden-and-build theory says that positive emotions broaden thought and action, enabling individuals to be flexible in higher-level connections and consider wider-than-usual ranges of precepts, ideas, and actions.
- It's important to develop new strategies to move our organizations forward in a digital era, utilizing new data and technologies as tools to fuel broader, more realistic, and richer views of our organizations and lives, thus having them be contributing factors rather than distracting ones.
- Positive emotions have been shown to help patients rebound from adversity, improve cardiovascular reactivity, ward off depressive symptoms, and continue to grow.
- Positivity ratio of three-to-one—it turns out that flourishing teams have greater than a three-to-one ratio of positive statements to negative statements in their meetings and interactions.

An example of incorporating the information:

- Person-first communication versus defining by disability
- Providing affirmation, for example, "You came to the right place."

- Establishing a connection that enables rapport
- Personalized instruction
- Personalized follow-up
- Choosing enabling words over those that trigger. For example, normative aging findings on an x-ray could be called "arthritis" or "wrinkles on the inside," but the former can lead a patient to believe they have something seriously wrong, while the latter may guide them to believe they are aging normally.

Chapter Three—Self-Efficacy

A few talking points listed as a reminder:

- Patients with low belief in themselves and low self-efficacy need someone who believes in them for the patients to be able to reach their goals. It is your job as a Called to Care provider to guide and encourage these patients along the way. If you believe in them, they will believe in themselves, too.
- Patients with high self-efficacy have higher scores on outcome measures when it comes to perceptions of function, pain, and belief in their own ability. So, improving your patients' self-efficacy is key.

An example of incorporating the information:

- The use of mental imaging can be very useful for patients in the clinic.
- Examples of previous patients who have struggled with similar problems but have come out the other side stronger than before are also good.
- Reassuring your patients that they are fine to do certain activities and decreasing their fear of movement through your use of positive language is another helpful thing you can do for your patient.

Chapter Four—The Art and Science of Positive Interactions

Active and Constructive Responding

	PASSIVE	ACTIVE
CONSTRUCTIVE	• Low Energy • Delayed Response • Quiet 🙂 *Cool.*	• Enthusiastic Support • Eye Contact • Authentic 😀 *That's fantastic! I knew you could do it. How did that make you feel?*
DESTRUCTIVE	• Turns Focus Inward • Avoiding • Ignore Speaker 😑 *Huh? Time to do your exercises.*	• Quashing the Event! • Dismissive • Demeaning 🙁 *C'mon, really? Don't expect to do that every time.*

A few talking points listed as a reminder:

- The beauty of positive emotions, broaden-and-build, and the use of self-efficacy facilitation and active constructive communication is that all these techniques create an upward spiral that gives patients the connection they need to experience tremendous benefits that accrue to their clinical experience and what happens to them when they leave the healthcare environment.

An example of incorporating the information:

- During patient/client interactions, allow for time to capitalize. Capitalization on events allows for:
  - Reliving and reexperiencing the event
  - Rehearsal and elaboration enhance the experience.
  - Memory access: you remember events you communicate about frequently.
  - Positive social interactions: you are perceived positively in the eyes of others, thus enhancing connection with others (validating and care).
- Facilitate the patient's recount of their positive experience:
  - Ask the five "W" and one "H" questions: who, what, where, when, why, and how. This allows facilitation of commitment from the patient, satisfaction, intimacy, increased quality relationship between caregiver and provider (also known as the therapeutic alliance), and trust.

Chapter Five—Goal Setting

Types of goals:

- Performance goal
- Learning goal
- Intrinsic goal
- Start goal setting from the future
- Choose hard goals

A few talking points listed as a reminder:

- A performance goal is the typical one we focus on. This is any goal that involves measurable performance and enables patients to have at least some control over associated outcomes.
- Learning goals are also effectively utilized in healthcare settings. These involve setting specific demonstrated outcomes based on understanding certain key objectives that provide context for predicting performance. Example: "Tell me what you now know about pain."
- An intrinsic goal is one set by a patient and not by anybody else like family, friends, culture, or teammates.
- All goal setting should occur within the context of a conversation with the patient.
- Hard goals require a longer commitment, greater attention, and more diligence.
- Findings show the pursuit of goals outside of a person's

comfort zone resulted in greater feelings of authentic self-esteem.

An example of incorporating the information:

- Imagine a middle-aged man who is currently taking blood-pressure medication. He would prefer not to take medicine if he doesn't have to. During a routine physical exam, he shares this with a nurse practitioner (NP). The NP begins some inquiry into the patient's ideal future self. She discovers he feels he is too young to be on the medicine, doesn't like the thought of being on it for the rest of his life, and wants to make lifestyle changes to attain his best future goal of getting off all medication. The NP comes up with the idea of setting lifestyle goals like eating a healthier diet, consuming less salt, and increasing cardiovascular exercise as these may help manage blood pressure in some situations.
- When you begin with the ideal future (in this case, getting off blood-pressure medication) and compare it to present-day conditions (i.e., contrasting thinking), you create motivation, optimism, and positivity toward making the goal happen.

Chapter Six—The Science behind the Placebo Response

A few talking points listed as a reminder:

- Placebo = "I shall please."
- Nocebo = "I shall harm."
- Placebo and nocebo are real psychobiological responses to healthcare interactions.
- We should confidently and boldly reinforce to our patients a vision of positive progress and eventual results.

An example of incorporating the information:

- Attempt to embrace placebo while negating nocebo. The conscious decision to use words that heal (non-threatening diagnostic terms) will enhance the patient's experience and potentially improve the patient's outcomes
  - Positive reframing
  - Shape expectations
  - Patient preferences
  - Encourage adherence
  - Avoid using negative words

Chapter Seven—Peak-End Rule

A few talking points listed as a reminder:

- How we remember our past experiences is almost entirely determined by two things:
  - The average of how the experience felt when at its peak (best or worst)

- How the experience felt when it ended
- This peak-end rule is what we use to summarize our experiences. We rely on the summary to later remind ourselves of how the experience felt. This, in turn, affects our decisions about whether to have that experience again.

An example of incorporating the information:

- Each medical visit could end with a "what went well" discussion, which ensures peaks are revisited.

Chapter Eight—Putting the *Patient* Back into Patient Care

A few talking points listed as a reminder:

- Calcification—exposure to the bad means calcification, or becoming numb to human connections and emotions, ensues and dehumanization can set in.
- Decalcification involves any type of routine, habit, or ritual that enables us to stop and remind ourselves that we are dealing with fellow human beings and restores connection and thus humanity. It is key for rehumanizing.

An example of incorporating the information:

- During patient treatment sessions, sit down with them

every visit and talk with them about non-health concerns to remind yourself they are unique human beings and you likely have shared experiences and emotions.

- The key to managing the calcification process is to simply avoid focusing too much on the objective details, facts, and figures that force you into dehumanizing your patient into a diagnosis.

Chapter Nine—Gratitude

A few talking points listed as a reminder:

- Showing gratitude for the things you have in your life is a healthy thing to do and seems to get the ball rolling toward other positive things in life, such as the perception of less pain, less incidence of depression, and increased life satisfaction.
- Among many techniques, keeping a gratitude journal has been shown to lead to long-term gains in happiness in general.

An example of incorporating the information:

- Showing gratitude toward the patient for choosing to come to your clinic specifically is something that is easy and appreciated by the patient. Gratitude, in return, is often facilitated.
- For certain patient groups, one of their home exercises

could be to keep a gratitude journal that they fill out daily or weekly. This will help with positive outcomes and serve as a reminder of specific accomplishments or milestones they can now be thankful for.

Chapter Ten—How to Begin Making Empathy a Daily Practice

Each intervention:

- Empathy
- Mindfulness
- Pause breaks
- Touch

A few talking points listed as a reminder:

- Mindfulness training really does five things:
    - It decreases mind-wandering.
    - It shifts attention quickly (i.e., it allows you to shift attention "in the zone" quickly).
    - It allows you to focus for longer, which is a critical skill for deliberate practice.
    - It allows you to observe your own mental processes rather than be swept away by them.
    - It provides an enhancement of executive function. It is a time gap between impulse and action.
- Include on-purpose, temporary, intentional breaks that

enable active disengagement. This will provide replenishment and facilitate patient engagement when you return to caregiving.

- A very light touch has even been found to have significant impact.

ACKNOWLEDGMENTS

This book would not have been possible without the help of so many people in my life who magnify my ability to get things done and make me look better than I am—and they do so willingly, humbly, and magnificently. Brooke McVeigh Mugavin is among the very best at project management and its execution. For her uncanny ability to track our Called to Care courses, coordinate workbooks, persuade hundreds of therapists across the United States to participate, and even get her husband, Dr. Mark Mugavin, on board immediately after medical school, I can't ever thank her enough.

Thanks to Marty Seligman for developing the Master of Applied Positive Psychology (MAPP) and challenging us to impact our spheres of influence and to James Paweleski for being such an astute program director. He, thankfully, accepted me back into the program after I temporarily dropped out. Thanks also to Leona Brandwene, my MAPP advisor at the University of Pennsylvania. She is brilliant, and I was so lucky to have her advise me on this research and content. Also, all my classmates at MAPP deserve special recognition for exemplifying positive psychology in their domain. Special mention to my good friend Bob Easton as well as the good doctors in the class, Jason Powers, Samantha Boardman, and Joe Kasper, and the incredible writer Emily Esfahani Smith. Many of the thoughts in this book were fertilized as Bob and I debated by his backyard fire in Pennington, New Jersey. Caroline Adams Miller was in the inaugural MAPP class and became a coach and friend of mine. It was her encouragement to translate the positive psychology interventions that are supported by empirical evidence to the healthcare profession and to attend MAPP, thank you!

My partners and co-founders at Evidence in Motion (EIM)—John Childs, Tim Flynn, Rob Wainner, and George Burkley—have always been willing to push the envelope in education and physical therapy. Without their flexibility, *Called to Care* would have been another great idea that did not come to fruition. In particular, Tim co-authored an article on the placebo/nocebo effect published in the *Journal of Orthopaedic & Sports Physical Therapy* that began a key conversation regarding communication and its influence on outcomes.

I also have to thank Daphne Scott, Andrew Bennett, David Browder, Jeff Hathaway, Bridgit Finley, Pat Wempe, Andrea Baumann, and Kim Mascaro. They were among the first in physical therapy to buy into my perspectives on this topic (i.e., my interest in research and rationales focusing on nonclinical factors of clinical success), and they supported me throughout the process. Also, my pastor and life hero, Kevin W. Cosby, continues to inspire me with the work he does daily for the wonderful people in West Louisville.

I also have to acknowledge and appreciate several groups of "dudes" in my life. First, and notably, a grid of great guys that have an ongoing conversation and camaraderie spanning thirty-plus years dating back to high school and college at Bowling Green State University. They keep me grounded, informed on all things Cleveland, and in laughter almost every day. The second group is an extension of my YPO Forum who challenge each other on the ski slopes, golf courses, and otherwise. Of course, the groups are rounded out by my non-golf, golf friends who have gathered every year for over twenty years and my neighbors and good buddies at The Barn. They know who they are!

Of course, this section would not be complete without a shout-out to all my partners at Confluent Health: their intrinsic motivation for success and complete commitment to clinical excellence **AND** service excellence **AND** care and compassion excellence have differentiated our place in the market.

Lastly, my adult life has largely been defined by physical therapy initiatives, projects, committees, conferences, travels, and businesses; however, it is naïve to think these things could have been accomplished without the unwavering support of my family and their unconditional love: Patty, Aaron, Angela, Lauren, Donald, Jonathan, and my first grandson, Levi—much gratitude.

ABOUT THE AUTHOR

DR. LARRY BENZ
DPT, OCS, MBA, MAPP

Dr. Larry Benz, DPT, OCS, MBA, MAPP, is a nationally recognized award recipient for his expertise in private practice physical therapy and occupational medicine and is a co-founder of Confluent Health and multiple other startup companies. A frequent lecturer at PT programs, national conferences, and MBA programs throughout the country, Dr. Benz has been on APTA's Advisory Panel on Practice and The Board of the American Board of Physical Therapy Specialties and is a past trustee with the Foundation for Physical Therapy and past chairman of the University of Louisville. He is the recipient of numerous business and physical therapy awards, including the American Physical Therapy Association's Private Practice Section Robert

G. Dicus Award, Kentucky Physical Therapy Outstanding Physical Therapists Award, and Ernst & Young's Entrepreneur of the Year for his region. His foundation is the co-developer of Jacmel Rehabilitation in Haiti, which can be found at PThelpforHaiti.org. Dr. Benz's current interests include conducting research and integrating empathy, compassion, and positive psychology interventions within physical therapy.